Nursing Law and Ethics

Other books of interest

The Law and the Midwife
R Jenkins
0–632–03629X

Professional Discipline in Nursing, Midwifery and Health Visiting
Second edition
R H Pyne
0–632–029757

Occupational Health Law
Second edition
D M Kloss
0–632–036516

Health Promotion: Concepts and Practice
Edited by A Dines and A Cribb
0–632–035439

Expanding the Role of the Nurse
Edited by G Hunt and P Wainwright
0–632–036044

Nursing Law and Ethics

Edited by

John Tingle

BA (Law Hons), MEd, Barrister,
Healthcare Risk Solutions Reader in Health Law,
Director of the Centre for Health Law, Nottingham Law School,
The Nottingham Trent University

and

Alan Cribb

PhD, Lecturer, Centre for Educational Studies,
King's College, London

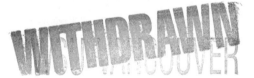

b

Blackwell
Science

First published 1995

Set by DP Photosetting, Aylesbury, Bucks
Printed and bound in Great Britain by
Hartnolls Ltd, Bodmin, Cornwall.

DISTRIBUTORS

Marston Book Services Ltd
PO Box 87
Oxford OX2 0DT
(*Orders:* Tel: 01865 791155
        Fax: 01865 791927
        Telex: 837515)

North America
Blackwell Science Inc.
238 Main Street
Cambridge, MA 02142
(*Orders:* Tel: 800 215-1000
            617 876-7000
        Fax: 617 492-5263)

Australia
Blackwell Science Pty Ltd
54 University Street
Carlton, Victoria 3053
(*Orders:* Tel: (03) 347-5552)

A catalogue record for this book is available from
the British Library

ISBN 0–632–03617–6

Library of Congress
Cataloging in Publication Data
Nursing law and ethics/edited by John Tingle
and Alan Cribb.
        p. cm.
    Includes bibliographical references and index.
    ISBN 0–632–03617–6
    1. Nursing–Law and legislation–Great
Britain. 2. Nursing ethics–Great Britain.
I. Tingle, John. II. Cribb, Alan.
    [DNLM: WY 33.1 N974 1995]
KD2968.N8N87   1995
344.41'0414–dc20
[344.104414]
DNLM/DLC
for Library of Congress   94-36996
                                     CIP

Contents

Preface

One of the key indicators of the maturation of nursing as a profession and as a discipline is the growing importance of nursing law and ethics. A profession which seeks not only to maintain, and improve on, high standards but also to hold each of its individual members accountable for an increasing range of responsibilities is inevitably concerned with legal and ethical matters. It is not surprising that these matters have come to prominence in nurse education, and enjoy a central place along with clinical and social sciences in the disciplinary basis of nursing. There is now a substantial body of literature devoted to nursing law and to nursing ethics.

This book is distinctive because it is about both law *and* ethics. We believe it is of practical benefit, and academic value, to consider these two subjects together. Put simply we need to be able to discuss 'what the law requires' and 'what is right', and to decide, amongst other things, whether these two are always the same.

The book is divided into two parts. The first part (*The Dimensions*) is designed to be an overview of the whole subject and includes introductions to the legal, ethical and professional dimensions of nursing, as well as a special chapter on patient complaints. The second part (*The Perspectives*) looks at a selection of issues in greater depth. These chapters contain two parts or perspectives – one legal and one ethical. The legal perspectives take the lead – the authors were invited to introduce the law relating to the subject at hand. The ethics authors were invited to write a complementary (and typically shorter) piece in which they took up some of the issues but then went on to make any points they wished. Thus the terms of invitation for the ethics authors were different, and more flexible, than those for the lawyers. This difference in treatment of the two perspectives is quite deliberate.

The essential difference is this: it makes good sense to ask lawyers for an authoritative account of the law, but it is not sensible to ask authors for an authoritative account of what is good or right – which is the subject matter of ethics. An account of the law will not simply be factual;

it will inevitably include some discussion of the complexity and uncertainties involved in identifying and interpreting the implications of the law. But it is in the nature of the law that lawyers should be able to give expert guidance about legal judgments. There are no equivalent authorities on ethical judgment. Instead nurses with an interest in ethics and philosophers with an interest in nursing ethics were invited to discuss some of the issues and/or cases raised in the first part of each chapter. Clearly these responses are of different styles and are written from different standpoints. Each author is responsible for his or her piece, and any of the views or opinions expressed within them. This difference between the two sets of perspectives is indicated (indeed rather exaggerated) by giving the former the definite, and the latter an indefinite, article – The Legal Perspective but An Ethical Perspective!

These differences in presentation reflect deeper differences between the two subjects. In short law and ethics are concerned with two contrasting kinds of 'finality' – in principle ethics is final but in practice law is final. It is important to appreciate the need both for open ended debate and for practical closure. When it comes to making judgments about what is right and wrong, acceptable or unacceptable, the law is not the end of the matter. Although it is reasonable to expect a considerable convergence of the legal and the ethical, it is perfectly possible to criticize laws or legal judgments as unethical. (This is the central impetus behind legal reform.) On the other hand society cannot organize itself as if it were a never-ending philosophy seminar. There are many situations in which we need some authoritative system for decision-making, and mechanisms for closing debate and implementing decisions – this is the role of the law. Any such system will be less than perfect but a society without such a system will be less perfect still.

Of course there are also areas in which there is little or no role for the law. The way in which nurses routinely talk to their patients raises ethical issues, and may also raise legal issues (e.g. informed consent, negligence), but unless some significant harm is involved these ethical issues can fall outside of the scope of the law. For example it is a reasonable ideal for a nurse to aim to empathize with someone she is advising or counselling; she might even feel guilty for failing to meet this ideal, but she could hardly be held legally guilty. Laws which cannot be enforced, or which are unnecessary, could be harmful in a number of ways. They could detract from respect for the law and its legitimate role, they could create an oppressive and inflexible climate in which no-one benefited. So even if we are clear that a certain practice is ethically unacceptable it does not follow that it should be made illegal. However the opposite can also be true. The overall consequences of legalizing something which many people regard as ethically acceptable (e.g. voluntary euthanasia) may be judged, *by these same people*, to be unacceptable – as raising too many serious ethical and legal complications. Both lawyers and ethicists have to consider the proper boundaries of the law.

Even these few examples show that the relationship between the law and ethics is complicated. Professional values, such as those represented in the UKCC Code of Conduct act as a half-way house between the two. They provide a means of enabling public discussion of public standards. They address the individual conscience but, where necessary, they are enforceable by disciplinary measures. We hope that this book will illustrate the importance of considering all of these matters together, and help to provide nurses with insight into what is expected of them, and the skills to reflect on what they expect of themselves.

Acknowledgements

We would like to thank Mr John Hodgson, Solicitor, Principal Lecturer in Law, Nottingham Law School, The Nottingham Trent University and Mr Harry Lesser, Senior Lecturer in Philosophy, University of Manchester for acting as editorial advisers.

Alan Cribb and *John Tingle*

List of Contributors

Ann Bird BEd, MA, RGN, RCNT, RNT, is Principal Lecturer in Adult Nursing, Thames Valley University.

Diana Brahams is a practising barrister at Gray's Inn, London and Hon. Senior Lecturer at the Department of Adult Psychiatry, St. George's Hospital Medical School, London.

Robert Campbell BA, PhD, DME is Principal Lecturer in Philosophy & Head of Humanities at the Bolton Institute.

Alan Cribb PhD is Lecturer in Ethics and Education at the Centre for Educational Studies, King's College London.

Alison Dines BSc, MA, RGN, RHV, RHVT, FWT, PGCEA is a Lecturer in the Department of Nursing Studies, King's College, London.

Michael Gunn LLB is Head of the School of Law and Professor in the Faculty of Law, Languages and Education at the University of Westminster, London.

Erika Kirk LLB, Cert Ed is a practising solicitor and Principal Lecturer at Nottingham Law School, The Nottingham Trent University.

Robert G Lee LLB is Development Director at Hammond Suddards Solicitors in Leeds.

Harry Lesser MA, B Phil is Senior Lecturer in Philosophy at the University of Manchester.

Jean V McHale LLB, M Phil is a Lecturer in the Faculty of Law, University of Manchester.

Jonathan Montgomery BA, LLM is Senior Lecturer in Law at the University of Southampton.

Reginald Pyne OBE, RGN, RFN, BBIM is Assistant Registrar (Standards & Ethics) for the United Kingdom Central Council for Nursing, Midwifery and Health Visiting.

G C Rumbold MSc, BA, RGN, DNCert, CHNT, RNT, DNT is Principal Lecturer in Nursing Studies at Nene College, Northampton.

David Seedhouse, PhD, is Senior Lecturer in the Medical Ethics Department of Psychiatry & Behavioural Science, School of Medicine, University of Auckland.

Arnold Simanowitz is a practising solicitor and Executive Director of Action for Victims of Medical Accidents.

John Tingle BA, MEd is a Barrister and Healthcare Risk Solutions Reader in Health Law; he is Director of the Centre for Health Law, Nottingham Law School, the Nottingham Trent University.

John White BA is Professor of Philosophy of Education at the Institute of Education, University of London.

Ann P Young BA, RGN, RNT, FRSH, MHSM is Senior Lecturer at the East London Business School, University of East London.

Part One
The Dimensions

Chapter 1
The Legal Dimension
Ann Young

'If he only knew a little of law, he would know a little of everything'.

Anon

Over the last ten years, nurses have become increasingly aware of the importance of law in their work. Their knowledge still tends to be patchy but it is now a topic that very much 'grabs' their interest.

Today's student nurses are also likely to be better informed on legal matters than previously. An 'understanding of the requirements of legislation relevant to the practice of nursing' [1] is one of the required learning outcomes of Project 2000 training. In giving care to the adult, child, mentally ill or mentally handicapped, an understanding of the relevant law not only helps to safeguard the patient or client, but also assists the nurse in avoiding situations with unwanted legal repercussions.

Law never exists in a vacuum. It is a reflection of our society and cannot be divorced from ethical and professional issues. Law always has to be developed and interpreted and the relationship between law, medicine and nursing is crucial in this process. Recently, legal cases on the interpretation of patients' rights and major changes in the way that the National Health Service (NHS) is structured indicate that an examination of the law as it affects nursing and patient care can become a commentary on the whole health care scene.

This chapter aims to give an overview of the interaction of law and nursing care. Section 1.1 examines the types of rules and legal processes that influence the nurse, from local policies, through case and statute law to European law. Section 1.2 looks at how the professional can influence the law. A vital component of patient care is working within a wider team of health care professionals and relatives, and legal issues of relevance to this are explored in section 1.3. Section 1.4 initiates some discussion of the knotty problem of getting the balance right between a nurse's duty of care and patients' rights. Finally, the effects of changing employment conditions on how the nurse functions are highlighted in section 1.5.

1.1   From local rules to European Community influence

1.1.1   *Policies and procedures*

A nurse's first acquaintance with rules that govern her behaviour is through local policies and procedures. For the NHS employee, many of these rules are enshrined in Whitley conditions of employment [2]. For example, the implementation of disciplinary action, the taking out of a grievance and rules relating to sickness are likely to have locally formulated policies in line with Whitley. Other policies are likely to have been formulated for specific groups of employees, for example, the wearing of uniform and the administration of drugs will only be relevant to nursing staff.

Such policies, while having their roots, some rather tenuously, in employment legislation, are locally negotiated and agreed. The usual route is for management to present a draft policy for consultation with the unions and, once amended and agreed, the policy becomes contractually binding on employees. A breach of a policy could then constitute misconduct, and resulting discipline could lead to dismissal if the circumstances were serious enough.

Some policies or procedures may arise directly as a result of legislation. Many complaints procedures were drawn up following the Hospital Complaints Procedure Act 1985, and the Health and Safety at Work Act 1974 and subsequent regulations led to a mixture of health and safety policies. Employees have trusted that local policies fully satisfy the requirements of the law in these circumstances.

Because of the contractual nature of employment policies, it is important that they can and are seen to be enforced. A policy that is unenforceable or commonly flouted is bad policy. Most nurses will be able to give examples. A uniform policy may be so unnecessarily detailed that little notice is taken of it and the reason for the policy long since lost. A drug policy may penalize the nurse who admits to making a drug error, leaving her less scrupulous colleagues to 'get away with it'. As the UKCC has pointed out, there should be a different outcome for the mistake made under pressure and the error that is the result of reckless practice [3].

A nurse's behaviour is also influenced by nursing procedures or practices, sometimes in the form of manuals or issued by a nurse practices group. These always have the status of guidelines rather than rules. The best of these are research based but the lack of sound or conclusive research material in nursing makes this an unattainable ideal for all practices. Even those purporting to have a sound research base should be examined carefully. The eusol debate seemed to be based on some assumptions as to the circumstances of wound damage with eusol. Disagreements between nursing and medical staff could, perhaps, have been avoided if the research had been better understood by both parties. However, case law supports the importance of nurses remaining up-to-date in their practice and this requires a sound knowledge base.

1.1.2 Case law

A major feature of English law is its interpretation through the court system and the resulting case law is of major importance to the quality of care received by patients. Any law can be tested in this way, whether criminal or civil law, or based on statute or part of the old unwritten law of torts, particularly negligence.

The law relating to negligence has been considerably refined through this system. The *Bolam* case laid down the principle of the standard of care being that of the 'ordinary skilled' doctor 'acting in accordance with a practice accepted by a responsible body of medical men skilled in that particular art' (*Bolam* v. *Friern Hospital Management Committee* (1957)). The *Wilsher* case (*Wilsher* v. *Essex Area Health Authority* (1986)) made it clear that the standard of care required was that of the post held, not the postholder. 'The law requires the trainee or learner to be judged by the same standard as his more experienced colleagues'. Although these cases involved doctors, there seems little doubt that these legal principles are applicable to nurses.

Case law has also helped to clarify the doctor's position in relation to death. In *Lim* v. *Camden and Islington Area Health Authority* (1979), and more recently in *Airedale NHS Trust* v. *Bland* (1993), the decision not to continue with treatment that is seen to have no purpose is well accepted. The Tony Bland case was of particular significance to nurses as this defined artificial feeding as treatment rather than nursing care, bringing it within the remit of previous case law. The interface between nursing and medical prescription has often been blurred and, although clarified in this instance, will continue to need teasing out, sometimes through the courts.

An essential ingredient of case law is legal precedent. In making a decision that is consistent with previous law, judges refer back to similar cases. However, not all decisions are binding on later cases. The case must have been heard in a sufficiently high court (See Figure 1.1). Thus most cases creating precedent have been heard in the Court of Appeal or the House of Lords, the latter being the highest court in the land and therefore overruling any decisions made in the lower courts. For example, the hearing to discontinue Tony Bland's treatment went all the way to the Law Lords in order to create binding precedent on all later similar cases.

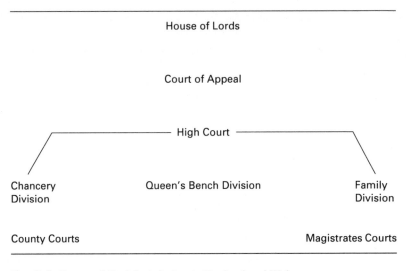

Fig. 1.1 Courts of Civil Jurisdiction in England and Wales.

In order to create case law, a case actually has to come to court. There are possibly several reasons for the paucity of legal cases involving nurses. One is the fact that the Health Authority or hospital employing the nurse is more likely to be sued (in the majority of cases where civil law is involved) than the nurse herself through the vicarious liability held by the employer for any damage done by the employee 'acting in the course of his employment' [4]. Secondly, employers are often tempted to settle out of court if there is an element of doubt as to the outcome. No court case means no case law and this can be frustrating, though understandable with legal costs so high, as it restricts the possible development of law in relation to nursing care.

One final point in relation to case law. For a case to be heard properly, there is a heavy reliance on the adequacy of documentation. An individual might not commence an action for negligence for up to three years from the incident or when any damage becomes apparent to the sufferer (up to 21 years or even longer for a child). With the pressure on the courts, the case may not be heard for several more years. Thus the importance of nurses keeping accurate and thorough records can be understood. The UKCC has issued *Standards for Records and Record Keeping* [5] to assist nurses in making adequate and appropriate documentation.

1.1.3 Statute law

Over the last fifty years, the creation of new law through statute has become increasingly important.

A number of these have had a major impact in the way that care is given. The Health and Safety at Work Act 1974 and the Hospital Complaints Procedure Act 1985 have already been mentioned. The Mental Health Act 1983 transformed the way that the mentally ill were treated and regular revisions of a Code of Practice as required under Section 118 of the Act ensure regular updating on advice as to the interpretation of this statute. The Access to Health Records Act 1990 has made nurses more aware of how they report patient care, knowing that patients can now ask to see their records. The Children Act 1989 has put the emphasis on parental responsibilities rather than rights. The Medicinal Products: Prescription by Nurses etc., Act 1992 gives community nurses limited prescribing powers.

However, these are only a few of the statutes affecting patient care and nursing. There can be little doubt that, for the nurse, the two major pieces of recent legislation are the National Health Service and Community Care Act 1990 and the Nurses, Midwives and Health Visitors Act 1979, amended 1992.

The introduction of market forces into the NHS through the 1990 Act has had a marked effect on how administrators, doctors and nurses work (see Figure 1.2). The business culture had already been implemented to some extent but the introduction of an internal market with provider units competing for contracts from health authorities has led to severe cost pressures. The resultant skill mix exercises have not been painfree. The setting of standards as part of the contracts should bear fruit in due course but currently the tools used for auditing standards are fairly minimal. Measurement of quality in nursing care, while easy for some dimensions, is extremely difficult for others, most notably those concerned with the psychological aspects of care.

The Patient's Charter [6], while not the law, does enshrine some legal

	HEALTH AUTHORITIES AND FHSAs		
commissioners	CONTRACTS		
providers			
GPs	NHS TRUSTS	COMMUNITY AND ACUTE NHS UNITS	PRIVATE SECTOR

Fig. 1.2 The internal market and structure of the NHS.

rights within it, for example the right to emergency treatment and the right to complain. However, there is some anxiety that some of the Charter rights may raise false expectations. The right to be referred to a consultant acceptable to you is rapidly becoming impossible if the consultant works for a hospital with whom the Health Authority does *not* have a contract for services. The right to be guaranteed admission for treatment no later than two years from the day your consultant places you on a waiting list has led to delays in putting patients on to waiting lists in order not to breach the two year requirement!

It has always been known that the NHS will never have sufficient resources to meet all expectations. *Re Walker's Application* (1987) highlighted this with the legal ruling that the Courts could only interfere if the allocation of funds by the Health Authority was unreasonable and in breach of public duty.

The legal status of nurses was hard fought this century. The most recent legislation, the Nurses, Midwives and Health Visitors Act 1979 as amended in 1992, allows the profession to regulate itself by 'establishing and improving standards of training and professional conduct'. Through delegated legislation, the UKCC is empowered to draw up Nurses' Rules that have the status of law once approved by the Secretary of State. Thus the profession has been able to implement Project 2000 training, the Post Registration Education and Practice Proposals and the use of the Code of Professional Conduct as a measure against which to judge misconduct.

1.1.4 The European dimension

The European Economic Community was established in 1956. The UK joined the Community in the early 1970s. The Community creates a common market; this is an area within which all the factors necessary to the economy (both the commercial and the public sector) can move freely. These factors are capital, goods, labour and expertise.

The member states of the Community gave the Community powers to make laws and rules in these areas. These laws take precedence over national laws which are inconsistent (*Costa* v. *ENEL* 6/64 (1964), *Macarthys Ltd* v. *Smith* 129/79 (1981)). The European Communities Act 1972 gives Parliamentary authority for the application of community law in the UK.

The scope of the Community has been gradually extended, most notably by the Single European Act 1985, which strengthened the common market and streamlined the community decision making process, and by the Treaty of European Union 1992 (Maastricht). This actually creates a new body, the European Union (EU), which comprises the states of the Community, but has wider political aims. The EU includes the Community (EC) and nearly all the law which applies in the UK is EC rather than EU law.

EC law is contained in the provisions of the Treaty of Rome, regulations made under it and the decisions of the European Commission and the European Court of Justice. All of these are directly applicable and effective in the United Kingdom (*Van Gend en Loos 26/62* (1962)[7]. There is a further category of EC legislation, namely directives. These were originally thought only to be instructions to member states to introduce harmonized laws by such means as the state saw fit. They bound the state but created no rights or liabilities for anyone else. The European Court of Justice has extended the scope of directives by insisting that the state and other public bodies abide by them (*Marshall v. Southampton and South West Hampshire Area Health Authority (Teaching) 152/84* (1986)), and that the courts must (as part of the state apparatus) apply them 'so far as possible' in preference to inconsistent national legislation (*Marleasing v. La Comercial* – *106/89* (1990)). This has led to considerable disagreement in the UK, as it requires judges to override the terms of Acts of Parliament, which they are not permitted to do under the British Constitution. It is however clear that, in an appropriate case, they must do this: *R* v. *Secretary of State for Transport ex parte Factortame Ltd* (1991).

EC law has had a direct impact on nurses in various ways. One objective has been to facilitate free movement of skilled workers by providing for the mutual recognition of qualifications. There are provisions relating to the general nursing qualification, but not to specialized aspects of nursing since these vary too much in scope across Europe.

Nurses have also benefited from the application of Article 119 of the Treaty of Rome which provides that men and women are entitled to equal pay for equal work. This requirement, whether used directly or via Directive 75/117, or as the basis for amending national law has assisted in reducing discrepancies in pay and fringe benefits. The Equal Treatment directive 76/207 deals with non-financial discrimination on grounds of sex and pregnancy. It also protects (predominantly female) part-time workers against indirect discrimination.

Most health and safety legislation is now underpinned by EC directives. The Lifting Regulations and the COSSH Regulations derive from specific EC requirements, and the latest general Health and Safety Regulations are also based on a broad EC requirement.

It has been suggested that 80% of current legislation is directly or indirectly EC inspired. These rules reflect a consensus of opinion within the EU as to appropriate standards. In many cases the existing UK standards either are the norm on which the EC directive is based or represent a very close approximation to best practice, so the effects are not very dramatic.

1.2 Professional influence on the law

1.2.1 Expert witness

The influence of professional opinion on the law is an important way in which law is developed. As was enshrined in the *Bolam* principle, the standard of care is that 'accepted by a responsible body of medical men skilled in that particular art'. However, as the judge pointed out in *R* v. *Arthur* (1981) a profession's ethical standards cannot survive if they are in conflict with the law.

The parents of a newborn baby with Down's syndrome did not wish him to survive. Dr Arthur, the paediatrician in charge, prescribed dihydrocodeine and water only. The baby died 69 hours after birth.

The case became famous as Dr Arthur was charged with murder, later altered to attempted murder as it was impossible to prove that the drug had caused the baby's death. A number of defences were established, one of which being that Dr Arthur followed established practice in his management of such an infant. During the hearing, an expert witness testified on Dr Arthur's behalf to this fact. Dr Arthur was acquitted.

An interesting postcript to this case was a small survey of 280 consultant paediatricians and obstetricians, asking what they would have done in similar circumstances. Not one of them would have acted in the same way as Dr Arthur [8].

Despite this question mark raised over the value of expert witnesses, their use is now often an important aspect of cases involving nursing care. Their use in cases involving back injuries has been instrumental in establishing the standards of training and equipment that an employer should provide.

1.2.2 Influencing the legislative process

A more obvious way that law can be influenced is through the legislative process.

In Act of Parliament officially begins as a bill. However, a number of stages may precede the presentation of a bill to Parliament. A Green Paper may be published by the government to test public opinion, followed by a White Paper which states the government's intentions in the proposed area of legislation. In 1989 the White Paper *Working with Patients* on the restructuring of the NHS was published without a preceding Green Paper, giving less time for public response.

There are two types of bill, the majority of which are government bills. There is a tremendous pressure on parliamentary time to take these bills through the procedures required for them to become Acts. It is therefore not surprising that the second type, private members' bills, are much less likely to become law due to lack of time unless the government specifically supports them. It is fairly easy for those against such a bill to use delaying tactics to ensure that the time allocated to debating the bill is insufficient.

The nursing profession can influence statute law in several ways. First, it is important that it gives a response to any Green or White Papers published and the format of the bill may well show some response to comments received by the time it reaches its first reading. During the progress of a bill through Parliament, further influence may be exerted by individuals through their own members of parliament. Finally, the profession has the possibility of persuading a member of parliament to put forward a private members' bill, although, as was stated above, the success of this route is limited. However, it can heighten public and political awareness of the need for legislation in a certain area.

Because of the time constraints in Parliament, much law is now enacted via delegated legislation, e.g. statutory instruments. As already mentioned, the Nurses, Midwives and Health Visitors Act 1979 functions in this way, enabling canvassing of the profession's opinions and discussion by the representatives of the UKCC.

It is important that, in order to influence legislation, nurses become more politically aware. The individual alone is unlikely to have much effect, but the government or Members of Parliament may find it more difficult to ignore a well organized pressure group. Unions and professional organisations recognize the importance of taking on this role but nursing still tends to be fragmented and lack a forceful united voice.

1.3 The wider health care team

1.3.1 *Working with medical staff and other health professionals*

The emphasis so far has been on the nurse as a practitioner distinct from other professionals. Of course, the nurse has never functioned in this way but the nature of her relationship with other members of the health care team is currently going through rapid change.

The medical and nursing professions have always worked closely together. However, it has tended to be a rather unequal relationship, the power being vested in the doctor. The law has largely supported this. The doctor diagnoses and prescribes, the nurse carries out his instructions. A failure to do so can lead to discipline or even dismissal as some nurses have found to their cost. Nurses have only been able to legitimately question doctors' decisions if they suspect negligence or criminal intention. For example, nurses are advised to refuse to give a drug if they suspect the doctor has prescribed a wrong dose [9]. To do so would involve the nurse in shared negligence. Similarly a nurse should avoid participating in giving a potentially lethal dose of a drug if she is concerned it may be prescribed to hasten death rather than for the relief of pain.

A number of factors are changing this rather paternalistic relationship. The increasing development and use of high powered technology in patient care makes it difficult to differentiate clearly between the doctor's and nurse's respective roles. Specially trained nurses are even becoming involved in carrying out minor surgery. The new general practitioner contracts put a heavy emphasis on screening and health assessment, previously areas of fairly low input. Doctors are finding that nurses are well suited to taking on these roles in the modern medical centres. On a more mundane level, the reduction in junior doctors' hours and the pressure on reducing costs lead to it being economic to use nursing skills in new ways, enhancing the nurse practitioner's independence.

With such developments comes increasing accountability. As was pointed out, the lessons learnt from the *Wilsher* case mean that nurses taking on these additional responsibilities must ensure that they are adequately trained and competent. Although there is a management responsibility here, the individual is the one 'carrying the can' both professionally and legally. The notion of 'extended role' [10] with its requirement for medical acceptance of the nurse undertaking certain tasks is a major breakthrough for the maturity of the nursing profession.

Government support for the implementation of the named nurse concept [11] has also supported this change in attitude. The use of this nurse to play a major part in co-ordinating the care that the patient receives is worth exploring. The co-operation of other health care professionals as well as doctors and social workers would be necessary. As the nurse is already used as a point of reference for many of these professionals, acceptance by the medical staff of such a role seems to be the only step needed. Surely the patient would be a major beneficiary from such a move.

1.3.2 *Working with relatives*

Relatives are the primary and most numerous carers of the ill and handicapped. Often unacknowledged, the role has been made more difficult by a lack of support from the very professionals who should be enabling them to function as effectively as possible.

Much of the care given has not been seen as requiring any particular skill. However, a brief review of the care normally given to the elderly and mentally infirm by their relatives will quickly highlight the fact that nurses are especially trained in these tasks, for example, planning appropriate nutrition, lifting and moving, skin and mouth care, reality orientation and occupational therapy.

More recently, parents of sick children have been taking on many more technical tasks as children are kept in hospital for increasingly short periods during their illnesses, and current thinking has been to involve parents as closely as possible with care. Thus parents are encouraged to give injections and care for intravenous lines.

With increasing awareness of the law, nurses are now querying the legal implications of relatives taking on care. It seems likely that in the hospital setting any care delegated to a relative should be with the understanding that the relative is doing this from choice and is shown how to do the task safely and, if necessary, supervised. In the home setting, it is accepted that some care is not specifically 'professional' although the offer of advice may be very welcome. However, for those tasks that are outside normal care that the family accept as their responsibility special training must be given or the nurse could be negligent in delegation.

1.4. Duty of care versus patient's rights

1.4.1 Duty of care

Lord Atkin laid down the basis of the duty of care that we owe to others (*Donoghue v. Stevenson* (1932)). A person must take reasonable care to avoid acts or omissions that he can reasonably foresee would be likely to injure a person directly affected by those acts. This concept forms a cornerstone of the civil wrong of negligence where a breach of duty with resultant harm constitutes liability and later cases have only served to refine this.

The plaintiff must establish three issues on the balance of probabilities:

(1) That a duty of care is owed by the defendent to the plaintiff.
(2) That there has been a breach of that duty.
(3) That, as a result of that breach, the plaintiff has suffered harm of a kind recognized in law and which is not too remote.

Fig. 1.3 Negligence.

There seems little problem in concluding that nurses have a clear duty of care to their patients. Indeed, nurses talk of being 'on duty'. It has occasionally been queried as to the nature of the duty when primary nursing has been implemented. It seems likely that the primary nurse 'off' duty has safely delegated that care to another nurse. Other staff and even visitors can also be affected by a nurse's behaviour and therefore she also owes them a duty of care although the nature of the duty is less intense as they are not so dependent on her.

From the patient's point of view, the concept of negligence is an important one. The patient must be able to rely on the nurse to take care to avoid harming him. An ill patient is vulnerable for so many reasons, from his illness and from unavoidable effects of treatment. His need for safe care is supported not merely by the professional behaviour of the nurse but also by her wish to avoid litigation.

However, there are several drawbacks to the patient's reliance on the law of negligence. Firstly, for an award of compensation, there must be resultant harm. This part of a case is often difficult to prove conclusively even when breach of duty exists. In addition, if harm is sustained, but *not* as a result of a negligent act, there will again be no award. The notion of no fault compensation has been suggested on a number of occasions [12] but it still seems unlikely that this will be introduced in this country.

A second difficulty is the inaccessibility of the English legal system to the majority of people. It is well known that the civil law is slow and expensive. As already mentioned, it may take years for a case to get to court. Legal aid is only available to those on a very low income and circumstances have been recorded of unsuccessful litigants losing their homes in order to pay their own and the defendants' costs.

A third result of the law of negligence can be defensive professional practice. Defensive medicine has been recognized as a possible response, and a similar situation can occur in nursing. Practices can become restrictive in order to minimize the risk of accidents and this is often detrimental to the proper rehabilitation of the patient.

1.4.2 *Patient choice*

As lay people become more knowledgeable about their bodies, their illnesses and possible treatments, they often feel the need to be more involved in decisions as to the care that they receive.

The law has always supported this wish through the law relating to consent to treatment. The roots to this are assault and battery. A legal defence against a civil action for battery is that the patient has consented to the treatment. Consent must involve understanding that to which the patient is agreeing. The debate as to how much knowledge the patient needs in order to have sufficient understanding has been debated both in and outside of the courts. Mrs Sidaway found that in 1974 she had no right to expect to be told of a 1–2% risk of severe damage during surgery as she was told as much as would have been accepted as proper by a body of skilled and experienced surgeons (*Sidaway* v. *Board of Governors of Bethlem Royal Hospital* (1985)). Other cases have also supported the right of the doctor to decide how much information to give.

The nurse can play an important role in this process. She can reinforce or clarify information already given, she can assist the patient to ask questions, and she can play a part in assessing how much the patient actually wants to know.

Playing the part of patient's advocate in this way is not easy. It can lead to conflict with the medical establishment and the nurse must be careful not to step into the doctor's shoes by giving information on prognosis about which she may not be well informed. There can be negligence in giving wrong information. She also needs to honour the patient's wishes even if they are contrary to her own views. A patient may decide to refuse life-saving treatment or willingly embark on a drug regime that will cause considerable discomfort with limited benefits. Such choices are the patient's right and the professional responsibility is in ensuring that sufficient information is given on which the patient can base a reasoned, even if seemingly irrational, decision.

Patients who lack sufficient understanding to give a valid consent, also have rights. Children and the mentally impaired may have to leave the decisions over treatment to others. In these circumstances, teasing out what is in the patient's best interest has become the key principle (*F* v. *West Berkshire Health Authority* (1989)). How this is decided must also be questioned. Although good practice may suggest consultation with all members of the health care team, the doctor is under no legal compulsion to do so.

1.4.3 Getting the balance right

There are a number of dilemmas in getting the balance right between the law on negligence and that relating to battery.

As already mentioned, the duty of care emphasizes safeguarding the patient from harm and can lead to restrictive practices. It also emphasizes the professional responsibility to act with a fear that an omission to give care may be interpreted as a failure towards the patient.

In reality there is plenty of scope for escaping from such legal confines. The notion of accepted practice supports allowing the patient freedom in spite of this increasing the risk of harm. The practice of risk management is an important one. The nurse needs deliberately to weigh up the potential harm and potential benefit of certain actions for that particular patient at that particular time, and reach a decision which is then documented in the notes on which action gives the most benefit and least harm. In the case of harm resulting, she can then argue logically as to how her decision was reached.

A legal dilemma also arises when there is a pressure on the professional to gain the patient's co-operation to certain treatment or care. It is tempting to slant the information given or limit the amount in order to gain the required consent. For example, patients have not always been told that they have choices when participating in a research programme as there is a pressure to have even numbers undertaking different treatments. This has led to considerable distress, and not just amongst the patients. A unit may also need to argue for continuing funding on the basis of numbers of patients accepting treatment. Not surprisingly, some professionals find the ethical approach required difficult to accept.

Recently, there is an increasing body of opinion that suggests that greater openness with patients does *not* cause the problems that the medical staff often fear. Patients are prepared to take risks, they can understand the difficulties doctors face in treating incurable ailments and they appreciate and co-operate with a partnership in care and decision making rather than paternalistic attitudes. However, old habits die hard! Both nurses and doctors must strive to have insight into their own prejudices and assumptions. There is still a lurking fear that the more patients know, the more they will leap to litigation if things go wrong.

1.5 Employer and employee

1.5.1 Changing employment conditions

The employment context in which care is given has an important influence on standards. The National Health Service and Community Care Act 1990 has provided a major catalyst for change and pressures to reduce salary costs in order to push down contract prices have resulted. The nursing salary budget is a large part of the total budget of any health care provider and is therefore receiving close attention.

For some years there has been a move to care for individuals in the community rather than in hospital. The mentally ill, mentally handicapped and elderly have been the main recipients of this policy. As a result of the 1990 Act, the responsibility for many of these individuals has now passed from the NHS to the social services departments of local authorities. Hospital beds for long stay care have closed with an increasing reliance on the private sector.

Within the acute sector, there has also been rationalization on a regional basis with some reorganization of services. The government response to the Tomlinson Report (1992)[13] requires there to be a reduction of hospital beds in central London and increasing investment in the primary care sector. The possibility of this pattern being repeated in other major urban areas cannot be ignored.

The nurse is therefore likely to face a variety of legal employment outcomes. Most commonly, changes to job content may result from reorganization as employers aim to make more effective use of staff. Where staff need further training to meet such changes, or in order to transfer to a different job, fixed term contracts may be offered to cover the period of training. Some staff will face changes in their contracts where there is a transfer to a new employer, with changes in conditions of employment if the new employer is not within the NHS. Finally nurses may face dismissal due to redundancy and/or reorganization.

1.5.2 *Rights and duties*

As in most aspects of life, employers and employees have both rights and duties. A large amount of statutory interference has replaced the previous *laissez-faire* approach towards employment situations. The creation of the concept of 'continuous employment' under the Contracts of Employment Act 1963 underpins a large number of employee rights, but of particular importance is the Employment Protection (Consolidation) Act 1978 in relation to unfair dismissal. With the implementation of the Trade Union and Employment Rights Act 1993 there is now no qualifying period for protection from unfair dismissal in cases involving assertion of statutory rights, for example the right to receive a written statement of terms and conditions of employment etc.

With the NHS, the application of employment statutes is seen as legitimate, particularly since the lifting of Crown immunity in April 1991. Thus employers have certain responsibilities not to dismiss unfairly and employees can take their cases for unfair dismissal to an industrial tribunal. Unions have certain rights to be informed of changes, but not necessarily to be consulted. For most NHS employees, the importance of Whitley terms and conditions of service cannot be underestimated as these more than adequately enforce the law through their link with the employment contract. Those Trusts that are now opting out of Whitley, may or may not provide similar conditions and employees are having to check these more carefully than in the past.

However, there has to be recognition of the right of management to reorganize and change the workforce as changes in the provision of care require. Staff need to be supported through the resultant uncertainties in order for morale to be maintained and patient care to remain good.

1.5.3 *Employment and accountability*

Accountability is not a word that is used within a legal context but is important professionally. Definitions usually emphasize responsibility for actions, being answerable and making decisions based on knowledge and understanding. Legally it is therefore a concept closely related to that of duty of care and negligence.

The position of the nurse in relation to the patients, their relatives and her colleagues has been explored. This section particularly highlights how changing employment circumstances can put pressure on the nurse and may affect her professional practice.

There is now clear support for the individual practitioner to make decisions to widen her role within the context of the changing environment. The UKCC document *The Scope of Professional Practice* [14] states that practice must be

'sensitive, relevant and responsive to the needs of individual patients and clients and have the capacity to adjust, where and when appropriate, to changing circumstances'.

This approach has been endorsed by the Department of Health [15] who state that

'each practitioner is personally accountable for her own practice and for the maintenance and development of her knowledge and competence'.

The debate therefore no longer seems to centre on whether the nurse *chooses* to undertake an extension to her normal role (as previously possible). There seems to be an expectation that she will adapt when required to do so. One side of the coin sees this as a very positive advance in the autonomy of the nurse but the other side must be concerned that the nurse is being put under considerable pressure to undertake new practices to the possible detriment of the care she currently gives.

The requirement that each nurse is responsible for her own development is also positive. But history has shown only too often in a variety of industries and services in the UK that where money is tight, training activity suffers. Whether the nurse gets supported, financially or with time off, to undertake further training and education will have to be seen. The difficulty that the profession has experienced in getting a statutory requirement for five days of study leave every three years under the PREPP recommendations does not bode well for widespread employer support of further training.

1.6 Conclusion

As well as providing an overview of the effect of the law on nursing practice, this chapter has more specifically attempted to identify some of today's issues that particularly affect how nursing care is given.

The changing relationships with other health care workers seem to be particularly critical when viewed in the wider context of the changing environment, politically, economically and socially, in which health care is given. The blurring of the professional edges, for example, nurse/doctor, nurse/social worker, nurse/teacher, must at some point lead to an examination of respective roles and shared learning and even the development of the generic health worker.

The climate of partnership between professional, patient and relatives is also having a major effect on how the nurse works. Promoted by the Patient's Charter and some recent statute and case law, the pendulum has swung quite a long way towards patients' rights taking precedence over the professional's view of the duty of care owed. Attitudes tend to be slow to change and the law can still be looked on to support a paternalistic approach, but nurses are in the position to play a key role in facilitating such a change.

Employment changes are putting considerable pressures on nurses. Many of these are creating exciting challenges for those able to respond but inevitably there are casualties. Change, continuing and large scale, is here to stay. It seems vital that training and education at both pre-registration and post-registration levels include the development of skills enabling nurses to respond positively and proactively to change. Patient care cannot but benefit from being given by flexible and adaptive professionals.

It has been very obvious throughout this chapter that an examination of the legal dimension of nursing, midwifery and health visiting practice cannot be done without frequent reference to ethical and professional considerations. The following two chapters particularly enlarge on these themes.

1.7 Notes and references

1. *Nurses, Midwives and Health Visitors (training amendment rules) Approval Order* 1989 No. 1456. London: HMSO, 1989.
2. Whitley General Handbook. London: HMSO.
3. UKCC *Standards for the Administration of Medicines*. London: UKCC, 1992. pp. 25–6.
4. See further Pannett, A.J. *Law of Torts*, 6th edn., London: Pitman, 1992, pp. 111–5.
5. UKCC *Standards for Records and Record Keeping*. London: UKCC, 1993.
6. Department of Health *The Patient's Charter*, London: HMSO, 1991.
7. See also Article 189 of the Treaty of Rome and section 3 of the European Communities Act 1972.
8. See further: Skegg, P.D.G. *Law, Ethics and Medicine*, Oxford: Clarendon Press, 1984. pp 147–8.
9. UKCC *Exercising Accountability*, London: UKCC, 1989. p 16.
10. DHSS *The Extending Role of the Clinical Nurse – legal implications and training requirements* HC(77)22 DHSS, London: DHSS, 1977 and Department of Health *The extended role of the nurse/scope of professional practice* PL/CNO (92)4 Dept. of Health, London: DOH, 1992.

11. Department of Health *The Named Nurse – your questions answered*, London: HMSO, 1992.
12. See Brazier, M. *Medicine, Patients and the Law*, 2nd edn., Harmondsworth, Middlesex: Penguin, 1992, pp 215–30.
13. Tomlinson, B. *Report of the Inquiry into London's Health Service, Medical Education and Research*, London: HMSO, 1992.
14. UKCC *The Scope of Professional Practice*, London: UKCC, 1992. p 1.
15. Department of Health *The extended role of the nurse/scope of professional practice* PL/CNO (92)4 Dept. of Health, London: HMSO, 1992.

Chapter 2
The Ethical Dimension
Alan Cribb

2.1 Nursing practice, nursing philosophy and nursing ethics

2.1.1 *The debates*

What are the values that shape nursing practice? This is a much debated question. Indeed most of the debate that takes place in nursing and academic nursing literature is about values. The only exception is debate about purely factual or technical matters.

Value debates take place about the nature of professional–patient relationships, and ideas like empowerment, partnership or advocacy. More specifically there are a host of particular debates about such things as how midwives can best protect the interests of pregnant women, or how far the work of health visitors should be dictated by the *Health of the Nation* targets. Set alongside these are discussions about the professional standards of nursing – the framework of which is reviewed in the next chapter.

All these debates should be seen as continuous with nursing ethics, because they all involve making value judgments about the means or ends of nursing care; in short they all ask 'what is good nursing?' Anyone who has an interest in, and some grasp of, these issues is already 'inside' nursing ethics although they may not have thought about their concerns in these terms.

2.1.2 *'Good nursing'*

This is not meant to imply that nursing ethics is easy – far from it – all of these issues are complex. In any case even if someone was very good at debating the nature of 'good nursing' this would not by itself make them 'a good nurse'! If nursing ethics is to be of more than academic interest it should have something to say about how people might become good nurses. I will return to this question later at section 2.7 but notice that there is some apparent ambiguity in it. If we talk

about a nurse being 'a good nurse' are we talking about her professional or technical skills or are we making an ethical judgement about
her character, or perhaps both? It would certainly seem odd to call
someone a good nurse if she could demonstrate many 'competences'
but lacked any concern or commitment for her clients or colleagues. In
this respect it seems very different from calling someone a good
mathematician; a set of skills which is, on the face of it, compatible
with being lazy, insensitive and self-centred!

2.1.3 *Nursing philosophy*

All nursing practice is necessarily informed, partly implicitly, by some
nursing philosophy. Such a philosophy embodies answers to a range of
questions which are faced by any nurse. These include questions about
the aims of care, professional–client relationships, working in teams and
with colleagues, and wider questions about institutional, local or national
policies.

Although nursing involves activities other than patient or client care,
such as health care research and management, it seems reasonable to
view care as central, and to see the other activities as supporting this
central one. But 'care' is too broad a notion to be of much help in
clarifying the aims of nursing; care is the focus, but what are the aims of
care?

An example of the debate about nursing philosophy and the aims of
nursing is what has been called the shift 'from sick nursing to health
nursing'[1]. The shift – which is dramatic in some areas of practice and
incremental in others – is from doing things *to* patients towards working
with them; from an approach which is 'disease based' and expert-
centred to one which is 'health based' and patient-centred. This shift
follows from and reflects many things, including changing patterns of ill-
health, emerging professional roles, an increase in consumerism, and
developing ideas about health promotion. But at its heart is what might
be called an ethical shift. A shift in values which has two interrelated
components.

Firstly, and rather crudely put, there is a move from treating people as
passive towards treating them with respect as equals. This is not only
because individuals have an important role to play in their own care, but
also because individuals 'deserve' to be treated with respect, whether or
not to do so is useful to professionals.

Secondly, there is a move from equating the best interests of patients
with being 'disease free' towards an acceptance that there is much more
to well-being. Quality of life, peace of mind, and self respect, for
example, are legitimate concerns for a nurse as well as disease management. These two components are closely related because one aspect
of well-being, an aspect which many see as fundamental, is being able to

make choices and have them treated with respect. These issues will be discussed more fully in the next sections, 2.2 and 2.3.

2.1.4 'Habitual ethics'

This example of a cultural shift shows the importance of what can be called 'habitual ethics' [2–3]: the ethical judgments that individuals make as a matter of course, the values that are built into ways of working. A shift in the philosophy or culture of nursing, which entails that normal practice and expectations are changed, has enormous impact. Practice can be enhanced (or made worse) for literally thousands of people. Generally speaking much less rests upon the prolonged agonizing about unusual and difficult cases.

Of course these sorts of shifts in normal practice are difficult to implement: they involve reform of policies, institutions, and so on. To reformers they might seem an overwhelming task, like trying to get the earth to spin on a different axis, yet they are the bedrock for any practical ethic.

2.2 Promoting welfare and well-being

Let us say, to use a piece of shorthand, that nursing is about the promotion of well-being. This seems a useful phrase yet, at the same time, it throws up a lot of questions. Many of the key ethical issues faced by nurses, and other health care workers, can be identified and clarified by working through some of these questions.

2.2.1 Well-being and welfare

Is this formulation of the nurse's role not too broad? There are many aspects of well-being; someone's well-being may be increased by a tour of the Mediterranean, by acquiring a new friend, or by learning Latin. None of these things, nor many others like them, seem to be the function of nursing. So perhaps it would be better to say that nursing is about the promotion of certain elements of well-being.

One currently popular version of this is to equate nursing with the promotion of health. This is only an improvement if we can give a meaning to health which is less all-encompassing than well-being, and yet less narrow than the idea of absence of disease which fails to capture all of the work of nurses. A number of authors have advocated such a 'middle-order' conception of health, with the intention that such a conception would help clarify the central objectives and priorities of health workers [4–5]. Broadly speaking these conceptions identify health with what others would call 'welfare', i.e., someone is healthy to the extent that they have the resources to pursue and achieve well-being or fulfilment.

In practical terms this would mean that nursing is about helping to ensure that individuals are in a position to travel, or to learn languages etc. This is not the place to review all of the discussions that have taken place on the theme. But it is possible to make a few comments on the central issues.

Although it is useful to try to clarify the aims of nursing there is no reason to suppose that a single phrase or formula will capture everything which nurses aim at. It is reasonable to assert that the central or overall aim of nursing is to contribute to welfare, but this simple formula needs to be qualified. Otherwise it is arguably both too broad and too narrow.

First, the way in which welfare is promoted is, in the main, based around the management (including prevention) of suffering or risk rather than wider aspects of welfare promotion such as financial assistance or education, although there is a place for these within health care. That is to say that nurses rightly do not regard the promotion of all aspects of all people's welfare as within their remit. They respond to the suffering of individuals, or to the risks faced by certain populations.

Second, once in a relationship with a client they need to have regard to all aspects of well-being that might be relevant to caring for that person. This is part of what is meant by holistic care, but it also follows from a concern with the promotion of welfare; for how can you know whether you are contributing to someone's welfare if you do not see what you do in the context of their whole life? Only by having regard to the whole can nurses ensure that their work is in the interest of their clients.

2.2.2   Costs and benefits

It is not possible to promote welfare, for example, without having regard to both the costs and the benefits of proposed interventions. Any intervention is likely to have some 'cost' or risk for the client which has to be weighed against the expected benefit; and there will be wider costs and benefits for others affected directly or indirectly. (We will return to this in section 2.4.2.)

2.2.3   Welfare and wishes

Neither can welfare be promoted without having regard to the wishes or preferences of clients. This is because an important part of my welfare consists in having my wishes respected. So even if a nurse is clear about her aims, and has a clear view of what is in the interest of her client, she faces a number of potential problems of fundamental importance. What if the client disagrees about what is in his or her interest? What if the client agrees that in some respects the nurse's preferred intervention is in his or her interest but for some reason does not wish the intervention to take place? What if the client is not in a position to express an opinion?

Under all of these sets of circumstances an appeal to 'promoting welfare' is not sufficient. A well intentioned intervention is not necessarily in the best interest of a client, and, even in those cases where it is, it may not be justified.

The possible tension between 'welfare' and 'wishes' is one of the key issues in health care ethics. Many of the contributions in this book discuss it in one form or another. How should nurses balance promoting the welfare and respecting the wishes of their clients? This is, for example, the background against which the importance of informed consent is discussed.

This issue is so important in health care because typically there is a patient who is in some distress and in a relatively powerless state and a group of health professionals in relatively powerful positions and who are charged with looking after the patient. Here there is a constant temptation to 'take over' in one way or another for the sake of the patient, without proper regard for the patient's wishes.

The ideal circumstances are those in which a client is able to discuss and understand the options facing him, and able to negotiate care and freely assent to any intervention. This assumes that the client is conscious, of sufficient maturity, mentally well and in an open and non-pressurised environment. When one or another of these conditions is not met then there is scope for ethical debate about how best to act. It is usually relevant to consider what the client would wish if they were able to express themselves freely. This might entail imaginatively 'putting ourselves in their shoes', or consulting their family and friends about their views. Sometimes health professionals or family members may be able to make an informed judgement based upon the wishes previously expressed by the client.

2.3 Respect for persons and respect for autonomy

2.3.1 *The value of persons*

Although it is certainly essential to take into account the views or wishes of clients it should not be assumed that it is always right for these wishes to prevail. What is needed is an ethical account of why 'wishes' are of such importance, and when, if ever, they can be overridden.

The intuitions which lie behind this judgment are so basic that it is difficult to produce an account. But the idea of 'respect for persons' – if we unpack it – helps to articulate it. In brief this is the idea that each of us has an intrinsic value which, if we are to recognize one another properly, cannot be ignored or 'traded off' for some other end. To treat someone only as an object, or only as a tool or resource, is to fail to treat them as a person.

This way of expressing the value of persons is derived from part of Kant's moral philosophy, and for many modern thinkers it is close to the essence of ethics. One way in which respect can be exercised is by taking seriously the autonomous choices which people make and not ignoring or overriding them. Hence the importance of consultation, partnership, and informed consent.

2.3.2 Paternalism

However respect for autonomous choices is not all there is to respect for persons. Parents may recognise the choices of their teenage children as autonomous, and may choose to override some of their children's wishes without necessarily being guilty of treating them as 'objects'. Indeed they may be treating them with great respect and love, and they may be motivated purely by concern for their children's welfare.

Acting in what you judge to be the best interests of someone else in a way that overrides, or limits the exercise of, their autonomy is called paternalism (or sometimes parentalism). As we have seen paternalism is a constant temptation in health care, and if we are to respect autonomy there should be a presumption against it, but are there occasions on which it might be justified?

There are two reasons why nurses may, from time to time, be justified in acting paternalistically. First, autonomy is partly a matter of degree. How autonomous a choice is depends upon a number of factors including the level of understanding and reasoning of the chooser. A choice made by a client may be judged autonomous at a minimum level, and as worthy of respect and serious consideration. Yet judged against a more demanding standard the same choice may be seen as not sufficiently autonomous to settle the matter decisively.

Second, it is often difficult to assess the degree of autonomy of a choice. Sometimes we cannot be clear what lies behind a decision or action, in particular how far it rests upon a misperception, a whim, a disturbed temperament, or external pressure. Under these conditions it might be justifiable to postpone a decision, or even override an apparently autonomous choice, in order to assess how far the choice really is autonomous. Both of these reasons are more likely to come into play if the risk to welfare is great (a suicide attempt is the paradigm case here).

2.3.3 The interests of others

Paternalism involves limiting a person's exercise of autonomy for his or her own sake, but there are, of course, other reasons to limit the extent to which what any individual wants goes. Respect for persons means taking into account the interests and wishes of all those affected.

Normally this means that the client concerned has the overriding voice, but this is subject to important qualifications. A patient or client, even if we assume they are 'fully' autonomous, cannot merely demand any intervention whatever the cost to other people, or regardless of the views of health professionals. If we are to respect persons, then nurses cannot merely be used as objects or tools to meet other people's demands – doctors or patients. This will happen unless they are involved in appropriate decision making, and allowed to withdraw in a responsible fashion from involvement when they strongly object to what is decided.

Also there is sometimes more than one client. A nurse may, for example, be supporting a bereaved family. Here respect for autonomy necessarily entails balancing the wishes of different individuals together, and having regard for the well-being of the family as a whole.

Finally a nurse acting as a budget holder or policy maker has to consider the overall implications of decisions for the general population.

2.4 Utilitarianism and the public interest

2.4.1 The dilemmas

This takes us on to the second cluster of problems concerning the promotion of welfare. How are nurses supposed to balance together the interests of different individuals, and how are they to consider both the needs of their immediate clients and a commitment to the general welfare or the public interest? A large number of practical dilemmas turn upon these two questions.

Dramatic examples of the first kind include those cases where individuals donate organs to others, or cases in which the interests of a pregnant woman and the fetus can come into conflict. Dramatic examples of the second kind arise when clients are a potential danger to the health or safety of others. If someone has a highly infectious and serious condition, or is seriously mentally disturbed, under what circumstances should they be able to determine their own lifestyle in the community?

2.4.2 Balance of costs and benefits

One way of thinking about these dilemmas is to see them as about totting up the expected costs and benefits of alternative courses of action in order to see which produces the best overall outcome. This way of thinking is called utilitarian, and there is a tradition of moral philosophy called utilitarianism in which it is defended as the basis of ethics. There are many debates about utilitarianism, and within utilitarianism, which cannot be summarized here. But it is possible to indicate both the plausibility, and some of the difficulties, of the central idea.

It would be odd to see ethics as simply about following rules for their own sake. Surely what we are interested in is bringing about better, rather than worse, states of affairs. A nurse who is asked to adopt 'ethical standards' will expect to see how they are connected to protecting or promoting welfare. Yet a rule or guideline which seems to work well most of the time may, on occasions, seem to do more harm than good. For example, it seems important to have rules to protect the confidentiality of clients, but it also seems that there are circumstances where the risks or costs of silence may be so grave that confidentiality could justifiably be broken. It appears that in this kind of example a more fundamental, and utilitarian, ethic is being appealed to.

However, there are some problems with this way of thinking. There is no exact ethical accountancy by which the different sorts of costs and benefits can be optimized, and different individuals are likely to disagree about when a guideline is unhelpful and can be broken. At the extreme this could lead not only to a climate of uncertainty about policy, but to a nurse's idiosyncratic conception of what counts as a cost or benefit having undue influence.

More generally a concern about utilitarian thinking is that it can involve sacrificing some people's interests for the sake of others, and that this could amount to treating people merely as objects or resources. There is, on the face of it, a tension between certain examples of utilitarian thinking and the idea of respect for persons.

2.4.3 *Resource allocation and ethics*

For example, consider resource allocation as an ethical issue which lends itself to utilitarian thinking. A nurse manager might have to decide how to divide a budget between a number of patients and the professionals who work with them. It is plausible to suppose that she should use her experience, and research evidence, to determine which pattern of distribution would 'do the most good' (although note the complexity and uncertainty inherent in this) and opt for this.

This sounds fine in the abstract, but in the real world it would probably involve overriding the views and wishes of the patients and professionals involved. Certainly any decision which entailed not treating certain sick individuals at all because money 'wasted' on them might be better spent elsewhere would appear to treat the former with less than respect.

For this reason many people react against utilitarian thinking, seeing it as 'immoral'. Yet health professionals, including nurses, have some responsibility to the general welfare or the public interest, as well as to the individuals in front of them, and need to explore ways of balancing these responsibilities.

2.5 Principles of health care ethics

2.5.1 The 'four principles'

One approach to health care ethics which has gained widespread currency is to set out fundamental principles, each of which needs to be taken into account when we make ethical judgements.

This approach, and the so-called 'four principles', have been made famous by the work of Beauchamp and Childress[6] and Raanon Gillon[7]. The four principles are:

- the principle of respect for autonomy
- the principle of nonmaleficence,
- the principle of beneficence, and
- the principle of justice.

In short, this means that in deciding how to act health professionals ought to

- respect autonomy,
- avoid harming,
- where possible benefit, and
- consider (fairly) the interests of all those affected.

This is not a formula for ethical decision making, rather it is a broad framework which can be used as a basis for organizing ethical deliberation and discussion.

2.5.2 Difficulties

There is no substitute for reading about this approach in the source texts referred to above. These make quite clear the difficulties in interpreting and applying these principles, and the ways in which they tend to conflict with one another in practice.

We have already seen that the idea of autonomy, and the ideas of costs and benefits, are open to different interpretations; and the idea of justice is, if anything, even more controversial. For example, some people would argue that a health care system in which health care is distributed by an open market, in which everyone has an opportunity to buy care, is perfectly just. Whereas others would see this as profoundly unjust, arguing perhaps that health care ought to be distributed according to need.

2.5.3   *The use of the principles*

This 'four principles' approach has come under criticism for being too superficial or too limited. Some of this criticism can be dismissed because it is based on false assumptions about the proponents of this approach. They are not arguing that all ethical thinking can be reduced to a few key words, or that the four principles provide a quick and easy method for solving ethical dilemmas. They are arguing that the principles provide a reminder of the key dimensions of ethical thinking, and that they can provide a common vocabulary and framework for individuals with different outlooks or philosophies. Although its proponents have produced sophisticated replies to critics this approach is, in part, designed to avoid the paralysis of endless theoretical debate, and to be of practical help in real cases.

Leaving aside the question of its ultimate validity, the practice of applying the principles to cases provides important lessons for nursing ethics. Although the principles supply 'rules of thumb' we cannot assess what we ought to do in a specific case without considering the particular circumstances of the case. Ethical judgment depends crucially on questions of fact as well as questions of principle, and it is worth noting in passing that a good deal of apparent ethical disagreement stems from disagreements about the facts.

Also because so much ethical thinking involves weighing together the conflicting demands of different principles it is possible for a small difference between two similar cases to result in apparently contradictory conclusions. We have already seen, for instance, how a decision to act paternalistically can rest upon very fine judgements about a client's degree of autonomy. Hence not only abstract reasoning but also sensitivity and attention to detail is an essential part of ethical thinking.

2.6   Philosophical ethics – its value and limitations

2.6.1   *Academic questions*

Philosophy students study 'Ethics' as an academic subject, albeit one which is normally seen to have an applied element. The questions typically considered in this context vary in their level of abstraction. The most abstract or general ones include, for example:

- 'What is the basis of ethics?'
- 'Is it possible to have ethical knowledge?'

- 'What is the meaning and the uses of the concept good?'

Then there are middle order questions which raise matters of practical substance but at a considerable level of generality, for example:

- 'What are the various conceptions of a fair 'society?'
- 'Under what circumstances is it permissible to break promises?'

Finally there are the most applied questions in which philosophers analyse the 'rights and wrongs' of specific policies or actions. In relation to health care this might include consideration of specific cases in which it is asked was nurse X right to Y (e.g. breach confidentiality) in circumstances Z (where these could be spelled out in some detail). Nurses who are also philosophers, or nurses who are interested in philosophy – and there are increasing numbers of both – will be interested in all of these questions, but what is their relevance to nurses with other interests?

2.6.2 'Selling' ethics

Philosophers who wanted to 'sell' their subject could offer the following argument:

> Every nurse has to answer the applied or practical questions, it is impossible to avoid answering them even if only by default (i.e. faced with circumstances Z you either do or do not breach confidentiality – you cannot fail to 'answer' the question merely by not thinking about it).
>
> But, it could be argued, answers to the applied questions lower down the list depend upon having or assuming answers to the sort of questions higher up the list.
>
> Therefore, if you want to answer the practical questions responsibly you must address the more philosophical questions.

This is a very plausible argument. It takes the same form as all sales talk – 'You cannot do what you want to, or have to, without my product'. For this reason we should be suspicious of it; however I would suggest that in essence it conveys a truth. The only way in which we can appraise specific circumstances is by standing back and comparing them with others. In so doing we will also find ourselves asking what kind of yardsticks, if any, we have. Are there some general standards we can apply, or does it vary from case to case, or from person to person?

2.6.3 *Standing back*

Philosophical ethics is a discipline which is commited to this process of 'standing back' and systematic reflection. There are a number of competing theoretical traditions which attempt to organize ethical reflection into systems of thought.

At their most ambitious they attempt to produce a single theory (or a unified set of theories) to account for all our ethical judgments. Given such an over-arching theory we could identify any particular decision, action, policy or person to be right or wrong, or good or bad, in specified respects. Philosophers disagree about the extent to which it is possible or desirable to aim for such general accounts, or whether they should be satisfied with the 'untidiness' of competing or complementary accounts.

They also disagree about the extent to which ethics lends itself to rational analysis, and the extent to which it is rooted in conventional codes and customs. (Note that these two things are not necessarily incompatible.) However anyone with an interest in applied ethics is interested in seeing how far systematic thinking can be of help in making or evaluating ethical decisions.

2.6.4 *Acknowledging uncertainties*

Hence one of the benefits of philosophical ethics is that it allows us to reflect in more depth about such things as utilitarianism, the idea of respect for persons, or the idea of principles of health care ethics. For example:

- 'What are the different versions of utilitarianism?'
- 'How far are utilitarian ways of thinking inevitable?'
- 'How far are they useful?'

We can ask these sorts of question in the hope that we might arrive at a definitive overview of the basis and nature of ethics, or merely in the hope that we will illuminate some of the complexity of the subject.

Although there is a danger that health professionals may see these philosophical questions as irrelevant traps (something like the four principles approach may be preferred as a 'working model'), it is important for everyone to recognize that these basic questions are hotly disputed – i.e. that there is no definitive 'knowledge base' in nursing ethics.

For example, in the health care ethics literature there is frequent mention of the value of 'autonomy' and there are many references to 'informed consent'. It would not be unreasonable for someone coming to the subject for the first time to assume that, in relation to such basic building blocks, there was a clear consensus as to their meaning and role. Thus it might easily be supposed that each time an author uses such an expression he or she is making use of a shared technical vocabulary; that, e.g. 'autonomy' always means precisely the same thing, that it is always valued for the same reason, and that its relative importance to other values is agreed.

In reality there are commonalities and differences in the way these terms are used, and this is not a product of poor 'co-ordination' but a function of the inherent contestability of ethics. (Incidentally some of these commonalities and differences are illustrated by the ethical perspectives in the second part of this book, and some disagreements about the meaning and value of autonomy are discussed explicitly in the ethical discussion of consent in Chapter 6.)

2.6.5 Other uses

There are a number of other things which the philosophical tradition can offer to nursing ethics.

First, there is a considerable literature in which the terms and issues of ethics are clarified and debated. Much has been written over centuries, and over recent years, about well-being and justice and so on.

Second, there are conventions for debate, based upon ideals such as disinterested and reasoned discussion, which can serve as useful models for people entering the subject.

Third, there are many issues of health care ethics which have philosophical problems built into them. For example, questions about abortion and euthanasia do not only turn upon factual matters but also upon intrinsically philosophical matters to do with the nature and value of life. In these cases it is impossible to treat these issues seriously without some consideration of philosophical questions.

Finally, and paradoxically, one of the benefits of philosophical ethics is an awareness of its own limitations. Being philosophically skilled is not the same as being a good person. There may be some philosophers who believe that a full ethical theory would be sufficient to determine what should be done in every set of circumstances, but no-one could think that this would be enough to make it happen. How would this perfect knowledge become embodied in practice? We all know that it is possible, sometimes all too easy, not to do what we regard as the right thing. For these reasons philosophers have to take an interest in character as well as in actions. What is it that makes people more or less likely to understand ethical demands, and to be disposed to meet them?

2.7 Being a good nurse

2.7.1 *Virtues*

One tradition of philosophical ethics, which is concerned with 'the virtues', sees these questions about character as being at the heart of ethics. The tradition is usually associated with Aristotle's ethical writings but it is a thread that runs through all of ethics. The idea of 'virtues' may seem old fashioned but it is a useful name for good qualities of character, in particular for admirable or desirable dispositions. To encourage children to do 'the right thing' we need not only to help them know what the right thing is but also to enable them to want to do it; preferably for it to become a habit or 'second nature'. The same goes for all of us.

It would be no exaggeration to say that nurse education and development is about the cultivation of desirable dispositions as well as the transmission of clinical skills. Some of these dispositions relate to professional attitudes and behaviour – such as research awareness – but underpinning them all is a disposition to care for patients or clients. The habit of paying attention to and responding to needs. Unless a nurse has this quality she cannot be, except in very restricted circumstances, a good nurse. And this 'skill' of caring is intrinsic to ethics. It is not like other skills which may be used in good or bad ways.

In fact caring is viewed by some as the pivotal concept of ethics [8]. Caring does not necessarily mean a self-conscious emotional empathy or identification; there may be many instances where nurses are too tired or stressed to *feel* caring. The whole point of talking about a desirable *disposition* is to make clear that an attitude which is rooted in feelings will persist even when the requisite feelings are absent.

2.7.2 *Changing virtues in changing conditions*

It would be an interesting, and perhaps useful, exercise to ask a group of experienced nurses to list the virtues necessary for nursing. At one time the Christian virtues of faith, hope and charity might have headed the list. Nowadays most people are likely to think of ideas like honesty or integrity, whereas ideas like patience or loyalty might be more controversial.

One thing is clear – as the conditions of nursing change a different balance of virtues is called for. No doubt humility is a good quality but as the pressures of individual accountability increase it needs to be tempered by courage and resolution. We all have some conception of what it is to be a good nurse. We can look at role models and try to identify which aspects of their character we admire. In this way we can set ourselves standards.

But this is not a sufficient basis for establishing good nursing. Individual nurses cannot be expected to pull themselves up by their own boot straps. Only the exceptional few could achieve high ethical standards in an unethical environment. It is essential that the cultures and institutions of nursing foster the virtues of nursing. This is why it is important to continue the shift towards a philosophy of nursing founded upon ethical commitments. This is why it is important to have professional values and standards articulated in public documents and policies. This is why it is important for nurses to be able to debate the underlying principles and the particulars of ethics.

2.8 Notes and references

1. Macleod Clark, J. 'From sick nursing to health nursing: evolution or revolution?' In: Wilson-Barnett, J., Macleod Clark, J. eds., *Research in Health Promotion and Nursing*. Basingstoke: Macmillan, 1993.
2. Oakeshott, M. 'The Tower of Babel'. In, *Rationalism in Politics*. London: Methuen, 1962.
3. Peters, R.S. 'Reason and Habit: The Paradox of Moral Education'. In *Moral Development and Moral Education*. London: Allen and Unwin, 1981.
4. Seedhouse, D. *Health: the foundations for achievement*. Chichester: John Wiley and Sons, 1986.
5. Nordenfelt, L. *On the Nature of Health*. Dordrecht: Reidal, 1987.
6. Beauchamp, T.L. & Childress, J.F. *Principles of Biomedical Ethics* Oxford University Press, New York, 1989.
7. Gillon, R. *Philosophical Medical Ethics*. Chichester: John Wiley and Sons, 1986 and Gillon, R. *Principles of Health Care Ethics*. Chichester: John Wiley and Sons, 1994.
8. Gilligan, C, *In a Different Voice*. Cambridge, Massachusetts: Harvard University Press, 1982.

Chapter 3
The Professional Dimension
Reg Pyne

Each man and woman who, following appropriate education and training, becomes a registered nurse, registered midwife or registered health visitor, also becomes a member of one of the regulated health professions. Their 'registration', since 1983, has been in the register maintained by the single statutory body established by Act of Parliament for these professions. Its title is the 'United Kingdom Central Council for Nursing, Midwifery and Health Visiting' (UKCC).

On 1 July 1983, this Council effectively replaced nine other statutory or training bodies which had existed by Act of Parliament or ministerial decision and whose powers (with the exception of the Northern Ireland Council for Nurses and Midwives) were concerned with one of the professions or with part rather than the whole of the United Kingdom.

3.1 The Nurses, Midwives and Health Visitors Acts 1979 and 1992

This change was brought about by the Nurses, Midwives and Health Visitors Act 1979, parts of which became effective in 1981 to allow the new Council to be established in shadow form and prepare for its future role. The Act came fully into operation on 1 July 1983.

The 1979 Act, having required in its first section that the Council be established and determined its constitution, goes on to prescribe the Council's functions. The Nurses, Midwives and Health Visitors Act 1979 has subsequently been amended in a number of significant respects by the 1992 Act of the same title. The 1992 Act reinforces the important principle of professional self-regulation which must be exercised in the public interest. It also disposes of a number of defects in the legislation and makes this important goal more attainable. The new Act came fully into operation on 1 April 1993.

3.1.1 The role and functions of the United Kingdom Central Council for Nursing, Midwifery and Health Visiting (UKCC)

Section 2 of the Nurses, Midwives and Health Visitors Act 1979 (as now amended in one brief but highly significant way by the 1992 Act) headed 'Functions of Council', makes it clear in its first sub-section that this legislation is not concerned with simply maintaining the status quo but with going forward in the public interest. Section 2(1) states that:

> 'The principal functions of the Central Council shall be to establish and improve standards of training and professional conduct for nurses, midwives and health visitors.'

Having nailed its colours to the mast in this way at the outset and established one of its major purposes, this primary legislation, in most of the remaining text, sets out the practical means by which the public interest is to be served by this statutory body.

3.1.2 Constitution and membership of the United Kingdom Central Council for Nursing, Midwifery and Health Visiting

In the course of the passage through parliament of the Nurses, Midwives and Health Visitors Act 1992, government ministers in both the House of Commons and the House of Lords made it clear that the principle of professional self-regulation was not in question, but would be strengthened by the amending legislation [1].

It is entirely consistent with this argument, therefore, that section 1 of the 1992 Act, which provides for the Council a completely new constitution, requires that two-thirds of the members of the Council be registered nurses, midwives or health visitors, elected by their professional peers through a democratically sound election process. Not unreasonably, given the government's obvious interest in the standard and quality of service provided for the public by these professions, the remaining one-third of the members are appointed by government ministers, this being done after widespread consultation with professional membership organizations, consumer organizations, medical organizations and others responsible for the management of health services and for higher education.

Section 1 of the 1992 Act simply states that the Council can have up to a maximum of 60 members and that the number must be divisible by 3, since two-thirds are to be elected and one-third appointed. Being sharply aware, from their own period of office, of the volume of work to be done, its 'public interest' importance and the demands of membership on people in employment, the members of Council prior to the reconstitution (with whom the decision rested) opted for the maximum size and proceeded with the election of members accordingly.

The position is, therefore, that the UKCC now consists of 40 registered nurses, midwives and health visitors elected by their peers and 20 other members appointed by government ministers.

In respect of the appointed members, the 1992 Act requires that the Secretary of State appoint from among persons who are registered nurses, midwives and health visitors, registered medical practitioners and others who are equipped to be of assistance to the Council in the performance of its functions. In making these appointments to the reconstituted Council for the membership term which commenced on 1 April 1993, making the decisions after the results of the election of members had been declared, the Secretary of State appointed nine further nurses, midwives and health visitors (several involved in health service management or in higher education), three registered medical practitioners, three 'lay' persons involved in health services management, two persons nominated by consumer organizations, two persons from higher education and one specialist in public finance and accountancy. Together with the 40 elected members, these members constitute the Council for the 1993–1998 membership term and, together with the Council's Registrar and staff, bear the burden of performing the functions prescribed for the Council in law.

3.2 The professional register

At the heart of the Council's activities is the register. This is not simply a large list of names with some associated details. It is something which the law requires be established and maintained for a very important purpose.

The professional register is, in effect, a means of declaring, to all with an interest in knowing, that the men and women whose names feature within it are those from whom a reasonable standard of competence and conduct may be expected. But it goes beyond that. It is also stating, in effect, that these are the people to whom the Council has declared its expectations, given its advice and presented its standards and whom it can call to account.

Since the introduction of periodic registration, requiring renewal of effective registration by individual practitioners each three years, the register, through the statistics published from it each year, has become a significant source of information concerning the registered nurse, midwife and health visitor workforce. It can therefore serve as an important planning tool for both professional education and service provision.

3.2.1 Admission to the professional register

Section 10 of the Nurses, Midwives and Health Visitors Act 1979 sets out the duty placed upon the Council to establish and maintain the register of nurses, midwives and health visitors and section 11 of the same Act establishes the criteria for admission to the register. It is self-evident that, in order that the register can satisfy the first of the claims made for it (that is, that it names those from whom a reasonable standard of competence may be expected), stringent conditions have to be satisfied.

Admission to the register is achieved through three methods only. These are:

- Successful completion of an approved course of education and training in an approved institution in the UK supported by evidence of good character.

- Original and currently effective registration in a member state of the European Community where specific European Community sectoral directives exist (i.e. for the parts of the register for Registered General Nurses and Registered Midwives.

- Where neither of the above apply, following an application founded on original and currently effective registration outside the UK, individual evaluation of the application and satisfactory completion of the requirements (if any) to establish knowledge and competence appropriate for practice in the UK.

At the point of admission to the register, irrespective of the route by which registration has been achieved, the individual practitioner is provided with clear information as to the Council's expectations of them, of the personal professional accountability which they bear for their actions or omissions and of the process by which, if the subject of complaint, they can be called to account by the Council.

3.3 The Council's expectations of registered nurses, midwives and health visitors

Earlier in this chapter section 2(1) of the Nurses, Midwives and Health Visitors Act 1979 was quoted as stating that:

'The principal functions of the Central Council shall be to establish and improve standards of training and professional conduct for nurses, midwives and health visitors.'

That is an amazing, but most encouraging sentence to find in any Act of Parliament. It must be extremely rare – possibly even unprecedented – for a sentence of this length in any such Act to contain the three key words 'principal', 'shall' and 'improve'. So the matters to which the sentence refers are not to feature a long way down on a list of priorities, but are to be 'principal' functions. The second of the key words is 'shall'. The primary law uses a mandatory rather than a permissive term, so the Council has no option but to address these matters.

The third of the key words is 'improve'. This primary legislation does not accept that the Council might simply 'establish' standards of training and professional conduct. It requires that the Council constantly 'improve' standards in both respects, recognizing that to do so is a mandatory and principal function.

Whether it was achieved through careful and deliberate planning, with every word weighed and the relationship between words analysed and co-ordinated, or was the product of beneficial inadvertence, it is both important and precious. It is so not only for the reasons stated, but also because it placed together, in a phrase, 'standards of training and professional conduct.' In doing so it provides a reminder that the first of the two – 'training' – is not an end in itself but a means to a particularly important end. It also reminds us that standards of the latter – 'professional conduct' – do have something to do with standards of the former.

This sub-section of the 1979 Act is stating, as principal functions, certain ends that have to be achieved. At section 2(5) of the same Act, in respect of professional conduct, this legislation moves from ends to means when it states that:

> 'The powers of the Council shall include that of providing, in such manner as it thinks fit, advice for nurses, midwives and health visitors on standards of professional conduct.'

This is another extremely important piece of the primary legislation. It makes it quite clear that the Council, being required to improve standards of professional conduct, is empowered to give advice to that effect. It also establishes beyond doubt the point that the Council, being required to maintain the register of nurses, midwives and health visitors, and also being required to consider and determine complaints against those practitioners alleging misconduct, has the authority to set out its expectations in respect of their professional conduct.

In these respects the 1979 Act, as now amended by the 1992 Act, is very different from the various Acts of Parliament concerning the nursing, midwifery and health visiting professions which preceded it and which were effectively repealed in 1983.

3.3.1 The Code of Professional Conduct for the Nurse, Midwife and Health Visitor

The two passages from section 2 of the Nurses, Midwives and Health Visitors Act 1979 which have been reproduced and elaborated upon earlier provide the background in law against which the UKCC has developed its key statement of the expectations which it has of practitioners. This is the *Code of Professional Conduct for the Nurse, Midwife and Health Visitor* [2].

The first edition of this document was prepared during the UKCC's shadow period of overlap with the former statutory bodies and released on 1 July 1983 – the very day on which that Council took up the duties prescribed for it by the new legislation.

That first edition of the Code was a document, the like of which the nursing, midwifery and health visiting professions in this country had not seen before. It immediately challenged the members of the professions named in its title to recognize the primacy of the interests of those they existed to serve and to address those interests in their approach to their practice and the manner in which they conducted themselves.

The Code of Conduct is now in its third edition, this being published in July 1992. Although there has been revision of the text, refreshment of the wording and the introduction of some new material, the claims made for this important document remain essentially those which were made for the first edition in 1983.

The Code now reads as follows:

'Each registered nurse, midwife and health visitor shall act, at all times, in such a manner as to:

- safeguard and promote the interests of individual patients and clients;
- serve the interests of society;
- justify public trust and confidence and
- uphold and enhance the good standing and reputation of the professions.

As a registered nurse, midwife or health visitor you are personally accountable for your practice and, in the exercise of your professional accountability, must:

(1) act always in such a manner as to promote and safeguard the interests and well-being of patients and clients;

(2) ensure that no action or omission on your part, or within your sphere of responsibility, is detrimental to the interests, condition or safety of patients and clients;

(3) maintain and improve your professional knowledge and competence;

(4) acknowledge any limitations in your knowledge and competence and decline any duties or responsibilities unless able to perform them in a safe and skilled manner;

(5) work in an open and cooperative manner with patients, clients and their families, foster their independence and recognise and respect their involvement in the planning and delivery of care;

(6) work in a collaborative and cooperative manner with health care professionals and others involved in providing care, and recognise and respect their particular contributions within the care team;

(7) recognise and respect the uniqueness and dignity of each patient and client, and respond to their need for care, irrespective of their ethnic origin, religious beliefs, personal attributes, the nature of their health problems or any other factor;

(8) report to an appropriate person or authority, at the earliest possible time, any conscientious objection which may be relevant to your professional practice;

(9) avoid any abuse of your privileged relationship with patients and clients and of the privileged access allowed to their person, property, residence or workplace;

(10) protect all confidential information concerning patients and clients obtained in the course of professional practice and make disclosures only with consent, where required by the order of a court or where you can justify disclosure in the wider public interest;

(11) report to an appropriate person or authority, having regard to the physical, psychological and social effects on patients and clients, any circumstances in the environment of care which could jeopardise standards or practice;

(12) report to an appropriate person or authority any circumstances in which safe and appropriate care for patients and clients cannot be provided;

(13) report to an appropriate person or authority where it appears that the health or safety of colleagues is at risk, as such circumstances may compromise standards of practice and care;

(14) assist professional colleagues, in the context of your own knowledge, experience and sphere of responsibility, to develop their professional competence, and assist others in the care team, including informal carers, to contribute safely and to a degree appropriate to their roles;

(15) refuse any gift, favour or hospitality from patients or clients currently in your care which might be interpreted as seeking to exert influence to obtain preferential consideration and

(16) ensure that your registration status is not used in the promotion of commercial products or services, declare any financial or other interests in relevant organisations providing such goods or services and ensure that your professional judgement is not influenced by any commercial considerations.'

Minor semantic changes apart, half of the clauses have not been changed. There is, however, significant change to be found in the remainder of the text. The incomplete stem sentence, out of which the numbered clauses grow and which they complete, has been revised. This has been done to dispose of the belief of some that accountability was either something that others could bear for you as if by proxy, or possibly an optional extra.

Further changes are that clause 3 has been strengthened by deletion of the words 'Take every reasonable opportunity to ...' with which it formerly began. Clause 5 is completely new text, emphasizing the rejection of a paternalistic approach to practice and the need to foster independence rather than create dependence.

Clause 7 has replaced the former clause 6 which, during the period 1990 to 1992, brought the Council more correspondence than the remainder of the text combined. The burden of complaint in that correspondence was that the clause failed to indicate that, in their practice, practitioners on the Council's register should not behave in a discriminatory way and should not be selective about the categories of patient for whom they were willing to care. The replaced clause 6 read 'take account of the customs, values and spiritual beliefs of patients and clients.' As can be seen, its replacement clause is more robust and addresses issues which are at the heart of professional practice.

The passage of the document concerning the environment in which practitioners practice, formerly contained in two clauses, has been separated out into three clauses. These (clauses 11, 12 and 13) address variously matters in the environment of care which might jeopardize standards, in which safe care cannot be provided or where the health and safety of staff is at risk. They are all directed to the key theme of exposing those things which create a situation in which the needs and interests of patients and clients cannot be met.

It can easily be recognized that this document is a statement to all registered nurses, midwives and health visitors of the primacy of the interests of patients and clients. The first element of the introductory paragraph, together with clauses 1 and 2 make this point very clearly. This emphasis is surely right. It is the case, after all, that those who become patients or clients of health care professionals do so at times of great anxiety, dependence and vulnerability, and have no choice in the matter.

Similarly, it can be seen that the Code of Conduct goes on to spell out some of the essential ways in which the primacy of the interests of patients and clients has to be addressed. These are concerned with attitudes as well as actions, with competence as well as concern, with respect for the uniqueness and dignity of individuals, with truth rather than pretence, with advocacy and with the exercise of professional judgment in an unfettered way.

It can also be argued that, in these ways, the Code of Conduct provides something of a set of professional values. Without a doubt it provides, for individual practitioners, a template against which they can measure their own conduct, knowing that the Council will use it in exactly that way if such individuals become the subject of complaint alleging misconduct. For those who decline to view it seriously for more positive reasons, there is, therefore, an enlightened self-interest argument for taking the Code of Conduct very seriously.

One other claim made for the Code is that it is, in effect, for registered nurses, midwives and health visitors, an extended definition of professional accountability. The text of the document is deliberately constructed so as to place the words 'accountable' and 'accountability' in the stem sentence which is then completed, each in turn, by the 16 numbered clauses. Though they are printed only once, these words are effectively there 16 times. Each clause is therefore presented as an element of what is described as 'your professional accountability' for which 'you are personally accountable'. The unavoidable nature of personal professional accountability is addressed in this way. The concept of accountability by proxy is thus dismissed.

Last, it has been claimed that the Code provides a central and quite seminal set of personal standards related to professional practice on which the individual practitioner can build. In this respect it focuses attention on the quintessence of professional practice and care.

3.3.2 *Elaboration of the Code*

The UKCC has chosen to elaborate upon some parts of the Code of Conduct through a number of other published documents. In *Exercising Accountability* [3], first sent to all registered nurses midwives and health visitors in 1989, it elaborates upon the general theme of the exercise of accountability in general, and then addresses certain key themes in particular. These include concerns in respect of the environment of care, consent and truth, and advocacy on behalf of patients.

The publication concludes with a set of principles around which to exercise accountability. This passage states that:

'(1) the interests of the patients or client are paramount;

(2) professional accountability must be exercised in such a manner

as to ensure that the primacy of the interests of patients or clients is respected and must not be overridden by those of the professions or their practitioners;

(3) the exercise of accountability requires the practitioner to seek to achieve and maintain high standards;

(4) advocacy on behalf of patients or clients is an essential feature of the exercise of accountability by a professional practitioner;

(5) the role of other persons in the delivery of health care to patients or clients must be recognised and respected, provided that the first principle above is honoured;

(6) public trust and confidence in the profession is dependent on its practitioners being seen to exercise their accountability responsibly; and

(7) each registered nurse, midwife or health visitor must be able to justify any action or decision not to act taken in the course of her professional practice.'

In response to evident need, the UKCC also produced a document to elaborate upon the clause in the Code of Conduct on confidentiality [4]. This document also concludes with an important set of principles. These are as follows:

'(1) That a patient/client has a right to expect that information given in confidence will be used only for the purpose for which it was given and will not be released to others without their consent.

(2) That practitioners recognise the fundamental right of their patients/clients to have information about them held in secure and private storage.

(3) That, where it is deemed appropriate to share information obtained in the course of professional practice with other health or social work practitioners, the practitioner who obtained the information must ensure, as far as is reasonable, before its release that it is being imparted in strict professional confidence and for a specific purpose.

(4) That the responsibility to either disclose or withhold confidential information in the public interest lies with the individual practitioner, that he/she cannot delegate the decision, and that he/she cannot be required by a superior to disclose or withhold information against his/her will.

(5) That a practitioner who chooses to breach the basic principle of

confidentiality in the belief that it is necessary in the public interest must have considered the matter sufficiently to justify that decision.

(6) That deliberate breaches of confidentiality other than with the consent of the patient/client should be exceptional.'

These two documents, possibly to be developed and incorporated into a more substantial volume on professional practice, are a natural extension of the Code and find clear authority for their publication in the 1979 Act.

3.3.3 Standards documents

More recently the UKCC has chosen to publish 'Standards' documents and, through this means, to indicate the expectations which it has of practitioners in respect of quite specific areas of practice.
    Published documents of this kind are:

- *Standards for the Administration of Medicines* [5] and
- *Standards for Records and Record Keeping* [6].

These documents, like the Code of Conduct, have been directly mailed to all practitioners with effective registration to ensure, so far as possible, that they are aware of the Council's standards in respect of these specific areas of practice.
    Another kind of 'Standards' document issued by the UKCC is the Registrar's Letter which it produced and distributed widely in December 1992. This document – *Standards for Incorporation into Contracts between Purchasers and providers of Hospital and Community Health Care* [7] – seeks to influence for good the context in which registered nurses, midwives and health visitors practise. By this means it is the intention that those who employ these practitioners will state their expectations that they comply with the Code of Conduct and take steps to enable them to do so. The intention is to help dispose of any conflict between the Council's expectations of people on its register and a reasonable employer's expectations of a reasonable nurse, midwife or health visitor employee.

3.4 The Scope of Professional Practice

One further published document through which the Council has stated its expectations of practitioners is that entitled *The Scope of Professional Practice* [8]. This also has been mailed directly to each and every registered nurse, midwife and health visitor.

The key messages to practitioners to be found in this document find their roots firmly in the Code of Conduct in general and the introductory paragraph and first four clauses in particular. This document also contains a set of principles which are as follows:

'The registered nurse, midwife or health visitor:

- must be satisfied that each aspect of practice is directed to meeting the needs and serving the interests of the patient or client;

- must endeavour always to achieve, maintain and develop knowledge, skill and competence to respond to those needs and interests;

- must honestly acknowledge any limits of personal knowledge and skill and take steps to remedy any relevant deficits in order effectively and appropriately to meet the needs of patients and clients;

- must ensure that any enlargement or adjustment of the scope of personal professional practice must be achieved without compromising or fragmenting existing aspects of professional practice and care and that the requirements of the Council's Code of Professional Conduct are satisfied throughout the whole area of practice;

- must recognise and honour the direct or indirect personal accountability borne for all aspects of professional practice and

- must, in serving the interests of patients and clients and the wider interests of society, avoid any inappropriate delegation to others which would compromise those interests.'

Whilst these principles, like much of the remaining text, could be regarded as a statement of the obvious, the obvious sometimes needs to be stated.

The Council's expectation of each registered nurse, midwife and health visitor is, therefore, that they will think about the scope of their practice rather than its limits or boundaries. This will necessitate each practitioner, irrespective of the professional post which they hold, giving careful consideration to their practice and the context in which they practise. The result of such an examination should be the identification of those activities which, if drawn into the individual's practice, would be to the benefit of his or her patients or clients. The natural corollary to this is the acquisition of the necessary knowledge and skill to provide a broader and more beneficial care.

The intention of all of these publications, as of other advice given by the Council's officers through the written and spoken word, both individually and collectively, is that the care of anxious, dependent and vulnerable individuals should be of a high standard and an appropriate response to their needs. The intention is that such care should be delivered by practitioners who are always striving to improve their own knowledge, skills and standards. The same principles apply to those practitioners whose roles are more concerned with the prevention of disease and the promotion of health. Professional regulation, in order to be justified, must have such a positive thrust.

The former stereotype of the nurse as someone who saw 'good conduct' as being compliant and submissive is no longer appropriate. The new model is that of a practitioner who sees 'good conduct' as being informed, skilful, honest, open, questioning and challenging, and able to extend the scope of professional practice to meet the evident needs of patients and clients.

3.5 Proceedings concerning the register

Section 12 of the Nurses, Midwives and Health Visitors Act 1979, as now amended by the 1992 Act, requires the Council to 'determine the circumstances in which and the means by which ... a person may, for misconduct or otherwise, be removed from the register'. Other passages within this amended section now provide the Council with the power formally to caution a practitioner or to suspend his or her registration.

These powers are a natural and logical part of a system established in the interests of the public. If the register is to have any real significance it is not enough simply to control admission to it and to provide advice and set standards for those whose names are included in it. It is necessary to have a set of sanctions, and approved procedures by which they can be imposed.

The purpose of these procedures is not the punishment of any individual practitioner but the protection of the public. In 1983, just two months before the UKCC had to take up the burden of professional regulation, its first Chairman, Dame Catherine Hall, in her opening address on this subject at a conference at the King's Fund Centre, said:

> 'I believe that the professional conduct function should be seen in positive terms – as one of the means through which a regulatory body, acting on behalf of the profession, honours the contract between the profession and society by ensuring that any member of the profession who has failed to meet the trust which society has placed in him or her is not permitted to continue to practise, or, if the failure has not been a serious one, is reminded of the standard which professional practitioners are expected to meet ...
>
> The underlying philosophy of the professional conduct function is to protect the public, to promote high standards of professional

practice and conduct of nurses, midwives and health visitors, to ensure that justice is done, and is seen to be done, in respect of those who are brought within this function ...'

Although the 1992 Act has brought changes in the legislation and widened the Council's formal powers, that statement of the philosophy upon which this part of the Council's work is founded remains sound and applicable.

3.5.1 The Professional Conduct Rules

Section 12 of the amended Nurses, Midwives and Health Visitors Act established the Council's powers in this important matter. The full detail of the means by which those powers are brought into play is set out in subordinate legislation in Statutory Instrument 1993 No. 893. The full title of this important document is *The Nurses, Midwives and Health Visitors (Professional Conduct) Rules 1993 Approval Order 1993* [9] and it is published and sold by Her Majesty's Stationery Office, London.

3.5.2 Allegations of misconduct

The law in the form of the Professional Conduct Rules first addresses the means of considering allegations of misconduct. Misconduct is defined in the rules as 'conduct unworthy of a nurse, midwife or health visitor.' It is open to any person, including fellow practitioners, to allege that the actions or omissions of any registered nurse, midwife or health visitor constitute misconduct in a professional sense and call into question the appropriateness of his or her continued registration status. If such a complaint is received by the UKCC it is incumbent on its officers to investigate that complaint, to assemble the relevant material and to present it for consideration, in the first instance, to what is now called the Preliminary Proceedings Committee.

3.6 The Preliminary Proceedings Committee

Figure 3.1 sets out, in outline, both the procedures that are followed prior to the consideration of a case by the Preliminary Proceedings Committee and the range of decisions available to that committee.

A significant percentage of the 'complaints' received by the UKCC and which require the consideration of the Preliminary Proceedings Committee are consequent upon guilt having been established in a criminal court. There are well established procedures for a wide range of criminal findings to be reported by the police or officers of the courts. Such reports form the basis on which cases then proceed.

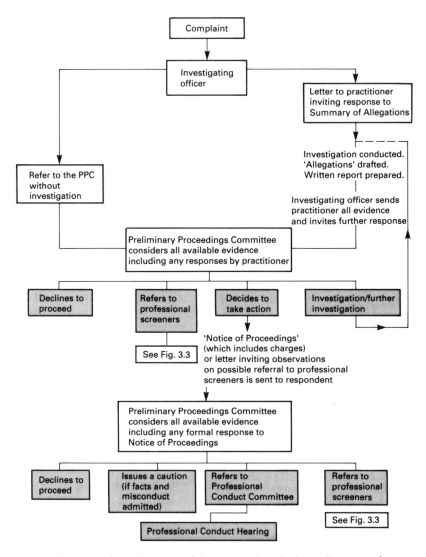

Fig. 3.1 A simplified illustration of the process by which an allegation of misconduct is considered by the Preliminary Proceedings Committee.

Where the complaint arises from an incident or series of incidents associated with a practitioner's professional practice, and which is not and has not been the subject of criminal proceedings, it is preferable that it be reported without delay. This helps to ensure that the facts will be fresh in the minds of potential witnesses and that they can be easily located. If a matter is regarded as serious enough to warrant an allegation of misconduct it should be reported immediately rather than eventually. Such complaints should not be delayed pending the completion of employment appeal procedures. The manner in which those proceedings are conducted and the standards of evidence and proof they require are different.

3.6.1 *The powers of the Preliminary Proceedings Committee*

As can be seen from Figure 3.1, this committee has a range of decisions at its disposal. If it believes that the facts or allegations (if true) with which it is faced are not of any great significance, or are unlikely to be regarded as misconduct in a professional sense, the committee can choose to do nothing and 'decline to proceed'. Rule 8 of the Professional Conduct Rules provides the authority for this decision.

If, on the other hand, it concludes that the fact or allegations are sufficiently serious that they will almost certainly be regarded as misconduct, and do raise questions about the practitioner's future registration status, it can refer the case for a formal public hearing by the Professional Conduct Committee. Rule 8 again applies.

A third option, newly available to the Council as a result of the Nurses, Midwives and Health Visitors Act 1992 and rule 4 is that, in certain circumstances, it can issue a formal caution. The Preliminary Proceedings Committee can only choose this option if the facts were established by a finding of guilt in a criminal court or have been admitted by the individual after consideration of the assembled evidence. A further prerequisite to the issue of a formal caution is an acceptance by the individual concerned that the facts are regarded as misconduct in a professional sense.

This new power seems likely to reduce the number of cases forwarded to the Professional Conduct Committee for hearing. In the past, the view that to do nothing gave the appearance of condoning a practitioner's unacceptable conduct led to many cases in which removal from the register was not a serious prospect being referred for hearing. This contributed to the backlog of cases and serious delays in scheduling. The author of this chapter had written of this prior to the passage into law of the Nurses, Midwives and Health Visitors Act 1992 [10].

If, at any stage of its proceedings, the Committee takes the view that the matters which have given rise to the complaint are symptomatic of illness or a consequence of illness it can refer the case to the 'Professional Screeners' in order that this view can be tested through appropriate means (see section 3.8).

3.6.2 *Interim suspension*

There is one further power now available to the Preliminary Proceedings Committee, to be used very selectively. This is the power to convene and conduct a hearing as a matter of urgency and to order the immediate interim suspension of an individual's registration pending an early hearing before the Professional Conduct Committee to consider his or her removal from the register. It derives from rule 3 of the Professional Conduct Rules. In the first year this new power had been used on three occasions as a means of urgent public protection. It is not expected that it will be used frequently, but it is an important addition to the means by which the Council can protect the public interest.

3.7 The Professional Conduct Committee

Figure 3.2 provides a simple flow-diagram concerning the stages of the process followed by the Professional Conduct Committee in considering an allegation of misconduct.

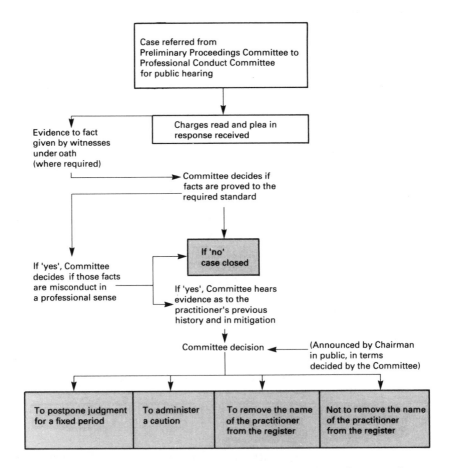

Fig. 3.2 A simplified illustration of the process by which an allegation of misconduct is considered by the Professional Conduct Committee.

The activities of this committee can be seen as the Council fulfilling its important regulatory and public protection duties in a sharply focused way. The ultimate sanction available to the Professional Conduct Committee – removal of a person's name from the register – is one of extreme gravity. It is therefore entirely appropriate that the committee possesses and, where appropriate, uses the power to sub-poena the attendance of witness. Similarly, it is important that the standard of both evidence and proof be very high. The standard employed in the criminal courts is adopted, so the committee must be satisfied to the degree of being sure beyond reasonable doubt that the matters alleged did occur as charged. Its decisions are exposed to challenge in the courts through appeal against a decision to order removal from the register or judicial review where a lesser sanction has been imposed.

To assist it in matters of law and to advise on the sometimes vexed question of the admissibility of evidence, this committee is required to have sitting with it a Legal Assessor. The law requires that he or she be a barrister, advocate or solicitor of at least ten years standing. The Legal Assessor is not part of the committee and does not participate in its decision making.

3.7.1 *The powers of the Professional Conduct Committee*

As can be seen from Figure 3.2, this committee's two extreme options are to remove a person's name from the register or to take no action in respect of the facts which have been established and which have been regarded as misconduct. Between these two extremes there now lie two other options.

Rule 18 of the Professional Conduct Rules provides the power to postpone judgment. The decision to postpone judgment for a period is, in effect, nothing more than a decision to put off a decision. It means that the respondent, having been found guilty of misconduct, is left on the register and left with the right to practise in the intervening period. It also means that he or she, at the end of that period must appear again before a committee which has kept open its option to remove from the register, and be the subject of at least two references concerning the intervening period from persons nominated by the respondent and who are aware of the misconduct proved.

It has been relatively rare to remove from the register at the end of a period of postponed judgment, but such resumed hearings that have been required have also contributed to the backlog and delay referred to earlier. This was one of the reasons why a new power was sought.

The second of the 'in-between' options is the new power, having established the facts and regarded them as misconduct in a professional sense, to administer a formal caution. The authority lies in rules 9 and 18. Whether issued by this committee or the Preliminary Proceedings

Committee, such a caution remains in the records held by the Professional Conduct Department of the Council for five years and will be used as antecedent history if, within that period, events occur giving rise to further proof of misconduct against that individual.

As Figure 2 also shows, this committee can refer cases to the Panel of Professional Screeners if it believes that the misconduct alleged is a product or symptom of impairment of the individual's safety to practise due to illness.

3.7.2   *Appeals and judicial review*

The two committees involved in considering complaints alleging misconduct, while not being deflected from doing their important public duty in the way they think best, must also be mindful of section 13 of the Nurses, Midwives and Health Visitors Act 1979. This section provides, for an individual who is aggrieved by a decision to remove him or her from the register, a right of appeal to the relevant Appeal Court for the country of the UK in which he or she resides.

There is no reference in the same Act to 'judicial review'. It is the case, however, that this widening area of the law has been used in recent years, by a number of persons who have not been removed from the register, to challenge the Professional Conduct Committee's decision to find them guilty of the facts alleged and of misconduct. The availability and use of the new power of formal caution might possibly lead to an increase in such challenges. In the majority of cases considered by the courts, attention has been concentrated upon the ability of the evidence to support the charges and the perceived severity of sentence. The Council's decisions have been upheld on the majority of occasions. Where this has not been the case the Council has sought to obtain from the judges some guidance on the element of the procedure which has been the focus of their criticism (e.g. use of the rule concerning rebuttal evidence) but this has not proved particularly successful.

3.7.3   *Restoration to the register*

It is open to any person who has previously been removed from a part or parts of the register to apply for restoration to the same parts. The rule relating to this procedure (rule 22 of the Professional Conduct Rules) does not allow such an application to be considered by the Professional Conduct Committee in the absence of the applicant. In addition to making a personal appearance before the Committee in a public hearing, the individual applicant must nominate as referees two persons with knowledge of the facts and who have known him or her since the date of removal The Council's officer obtains these references directly from the referees, having first advised them of the facts and misconduct proved. The Committee's decision is to either accept or reject the application.

3.8 Unfitness to practise due to illness

It has been explained, in the passages of text concerning the Preliminary Proceedings Committee and the Professional Conduct Committee, that they, if believing that the issue is possibly one of illness rather than misconduct, can refer a case for that to be considered and tested.

These are not the only sources from which such cases emerge. Just as it is open to any person to bring an allegation of misconduct to the Council, so it is open to them to bring their concerns about people who they consider to be unsafe to practise due to illness. A significant majority of cases come from such direct referrals. Rules 29 to 48 of the Professional Conduct Rules set out the procedures which apply in this area of activity.

Figure 3.3 provides an outline of the whole process. At the heart of that process is the opportunity to invite practitioners to be examined by two medical examiners of the Council's choice who have no connection with their places of work or locality and can approach the examination with complete objectivity.

3.8.1 *Panel of Professional Screeners*

Like the 'professional conduct' mechanism, these procedures operate through two committees. The first is the Panel of Professional Screeners. The figure indicates that this committee can, where it believes it appropriate, and where it believes that the issue may, after all, be one of misconduct, refer cases back to the Preliminary Proceedings Committee or Professional Conduct Committee, depending on its source of referral.

3.8.2 *The Health Committee*

The issue which the Health Committee has to consider is whether it considers the practitioner's fitness to practise as being seriously impaired by a physical or mental condition. If it determines that fitness is so impaired the committee has no option. It must prevent that practitioner practising by either removal or suspension from the register.

The effect of these differently worded decisions is the same – the practitioner is prevented from practising. The difference is important, however, and not merely semantic. Prior to the passage of the 1992 Nurses, Midwives and Health Visitors Act, the law allowed only 'removal from the register' as a means of public protection. The UKCC took the view that, while 'removal from the register' was an appropriate term to

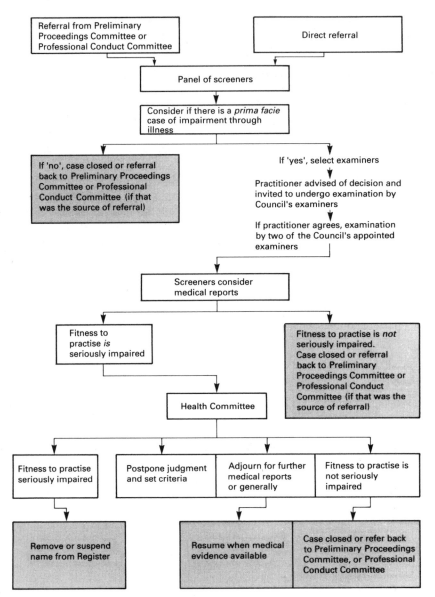

Fig. 3.3 A simplified illustration of the process by which complaints alleging unfitness to practise are considered.

use in respect of a person found guilty of misconduct, a less stigmatizing term needed to be used in respect of those who need to be prevented from practising, but because of illness. It seems likely that the Health Committee will 'suspend' registration, while the Professional Conduct

Committee will continue to 'remove from the register'. The latter committee does, however, possess the power to suspend registration.

3.9   The concept of profession

At the heart of any occupational group which seeks to espouse the term 'profession' must be clarity about the reason for which its members have acquired the special knowledge and skills that are regarded as essential prerequisites to practice. Knowledge and skill alone, however, are not sufficient. They must be supplemented by a set of corporate values, an appreciation of the meaning of accountability and acceptance of the importance of an ethical approach to practice.

The law described in this chapter, the precise duties which that law imposes upon the UKCC and the procedures through which those duties are carried out only provide part of the story. Control over admission to the professional register, the register itself and the power to remove practitioners from the register undoubtedly afford some protection to those whose interests these things have been introduced to serve. In order that those interests can be adequately addressed, however, these things must be employed in a very positive way by a statutory body which is never satisfied with its achievements. For professional regulation to have true meaning it must be exercised by a regulatory body which is clear about its important public service role and functions and conveys that clarity to its practitioners.

The presence of the word 'improve' in section 2(1) of the 1979 Act must surely mean 'constantly improve', rather than just go through one phase of improvement and then settle on a new plateau. Perpetual improvement, expressed in the particular context of each individual's practice, is something that can only be achieved by them as individuals. The UKCC can set the scene, provide the advice, guidance and standards, and set out the principles, but the professional judgments have to be made by each and every registered nurse, midwife and health visitor.

For this reason, in order that the primacy of the interests of patients and clients really can be served, the people whose names feature on the register which the UKCC, in compliance with the law, maintains, must possess and demonstrate important qualities.

It could take another chapter to set them out in full and elaborate upon them adequately. I simply close this chapter with the contention that they include integrity, honesty, determination and a clear recognition of the key duty of care that each practitioner bears. Add to these the relevant knowledge and skill and a necessary degree of positive restlessness, and I believe that nurses, midwives and health visitors, being members of regulated professions with a solid background in primary and subordinate law, are required to demonstrate that George

Bernard Shaw [11] was wrong in his contention that 'All professions are a conspiracy against the laity.'

3.10 Notes and references

1. Hansard, House of Commons, 13 January 1992.
2. UKCC *The Code of Professional Conduct for the Nurse, Midwife and Health Visitor*, 3rd edn., London: UKCC, 1992.
3. UKCC *'Exercising Accountability'*, London: UKCC, 1989.
4. UKCC *'Confidentiality'*, London: UKCC, 1987
5. UKCC *'Standards for the Administration of Medicines'*, London: UKCC, 1992
6. UKCC *'Standards for Records and Record Keeping'*, London: UKCC, 1993.
7. UKCC *'Standards for Incorporation into Contracts for Hospital and Community Health Care Services'*, Registrar's Letter 37/1992, London: UKCC, 1992.
8. UKCC *'The Scope of Professional Practice'*, London: UKCC, 1992.
9. *The Nurses, Midwives and Health Visitors (Professional Conduct) Rules 1993*. Approval Order 1993. S.I. 1993 No. 893, London, HMSO, 1993.
10. Pyne, R.H. *'Professional Discipline in Nursing, Midwifery and Health Visiting'*, Oxford: Blackwell Science Ltd, 1991.
11. 'All professions are a conspiracy against the laity', George Bernard Shaw, The Doctor's Dilemma (1906). Harmondsworth, Penguin, 1975.

Chapter 4
Patient Complaints in Health Care Provision
Arnold Simanowitz

4.1 Introduction

Anyone who has become involved with or interested in health care in the last five or even ten years might be forgiven for believing that complaints about health care provision have only become a real problem during that time.

Bodies such as the Community Health Councils, Action for Victims of Medical Accidents (AVMA), the College of Health, the Patients Association and the National Consumer Council have been vociferous about the problems and the need for change and even the healthcarers themselves have been admitting that all is not well for some little while.

The fact is, however, that the issue of complaints has been a serious problem for a very long time. As long ago as the 1970s it was so important that the government set up a special committee to look into it. The Davies Committee reported in 1973 and anyone closely involved with the issue of complaints today will be saddened to realise that Davies was able to identify problems 20 years ago which, notwithstanding the proposals then made to deal with them [1], have continued to bedevil the health scene ever since.

The difficulties for a patient wanting to complain are numerous and they will be dealt with in detail shortly. They all flow, however, from the fact that, in general, healthcarers have regarded complaints simply as a slur on their ability or performance and have therefore been unwilling to look at them sympathetically. It is suggested that this applies in particular to doctors, who have in the past colluded with patients to place themselves in a godlike position where the very idea of a complaint is unthinkable.

Any admission by doctors of fault of any kind was seen as undermining their authoritative position which it was universally believed was essential to maintain in the interests of the patients themselves.

Although the response by different groups of healthcarers has been the same, the reasons for that response has been very different although

59

not always identifiable. Those most at fault have always appeared, from the patient's point of view, to be the consultants. All organizations dealing with dissatisfied patients will have heard repeated stories about the arrogance of consultants, their unwillingness to explain what has happened or even on many occasions to make contact with a patient who wishes to complain.

That is not to say that there are no consultants who behave differently. There have always been consultants who have been only too willing to help and in recent years their number has increased. Nevertheless the old attitudes still remain with the overwhelming majority of consultants. Often the reason advanced for this by those who speak on behalf of the medical profession is the fear of litigation. In truth it is both the attitude mentioned above and a failure in the training of doctors which leaves them unable or unwilling to communicate with the patient other than about the technical matters in which they regard themselves as experts.

GPs are not obviously guilty of the same attitudes yet in some ways are more culpable. They usually have a closer relationship with the patient and the patient often relies on them to explain things where the consultant has failed to do so. What motivates a GP, who knows that a consultant has been guilty of a mistake, to forbear from telling the patient and often allow them to go for years without having a complaint resolved?

It is, however, often the nursing staff who are placed in the most invidious position. Trained for years to have loyalty to the team if not to the consultant, what is their position when something goes wrong? So often the story is that they will keep their distance from the patient or not engage in conversation in order to avoid admitting that the patient has suffered unnecessarily. What is their duty in that situation? I would suggest that their duty lies first and foremost to the patient. And today the Patient's Charter makes that clear. See the introductory letter to the Patient's Charter by William Waldegrave then Secretary of State for Health:

'This means a service that . . . always puts the patient first.'

Before the Patient's Charter, however, the UKCC *Code of Professional Conduct for the Nurse, Midwife and Health Visitor* [2] had spelled out clearly where the nurse practitioner's duty lay:

'As a registered nurse, midwife or health visitor, you are personally accountable for your practice and, in the exercise of your professional accountability, must:

(1) act always in such a manner as to promote and safeguard the interests and well-being of patients and clients;

(2) ensure that no action or omission on your part, or within your sphere of responsibility is detrimental to the interests, condition or safety of patients and clients . . .'

Lest there be any doubt as to the implications of those two paragraphs, the advisory document *Exercising Accountability* issued by the UKCC [3] dispels that doubt:

'The primary interests of the public and patient or client provide the first theme of the Code and establish the point that, in determining his or her approach to professional practice, the individual nurse, midwife or health visitor should recognise that the interests of public and patient must predominate over those of practitioner and profession.'

One of the most interesting aspects of these two documents is the use of the words 'accountable' and accountability'. For a decade there has been a demand from patients for the health care professions to be made accountable. As we shall see, simply putting the words into a code of conduct will not overnight make professionals accountable, still less behave in such a way that indicates a recognition that they are accountable. Nevertheless, once accountability is enshrined in a code of conduct the influence of that code, if it is enforced, will eventually have an impact on attitudes.

The contrast with the medical profession is stark. Nowhere in the doctors' code does the word accountability appear. The experience and evidence of patients is that it does not exist. It is for this reason that it is suggested that the nurse is placed in an invidious position.

What will the attitude of the consultant, and still worse the managers, be if the nurse who has witnessed something untoward offers the information to the patient out of concern for the patient's welfare and adherence to his or her own code?

It is these attitudes on the part of the health care professionals which led, first to the need to set up formal complaints procedures and then to their failure. What is not appreciated by many, or perhaps simply not acknowledged, is that whatever system is established for complaints will fail unless those administering it are committed not simply to the need for such a system but to making it work. It is for that reason that those outside the health service now believe that only a totally independent system for those complaints that cannot be resolved by conciliation would be likely to succeed.

4.2 The systems

If someone of negative intent had sat down to create a system for patients to complain about health care they would have been unlikely to have come up with anything as unhelpful as the present system, if that is what it can be called. Firstly there is an entirely different procedure depending on where the treatment takes place: if in a hospital then the procedure under Health Circular (81) 5 applies [4]; if in a GP's surgery then the complaint must be to the Family Health Services Authority (FHSA); and of course the procedure is totally different in each case.

There is a further distinction depending on the nature of the complaint: if it is about administration then the complaint should be made to the Health Service Commissioner, who also has jurisdiction if the complaint is about the way the complaint is dealt with – but not if it relates to a GP complaint.

If it is about treatment in a hospital then Health Circular (81)5 applies which can lead to an independent professional review by independent consultants – but not if there is or may be an allegation of negligence which might be the subject of litigation, in which case the independent review cannot take place.

If all this is not sufficiently confusing for the patient with a complaint, not only does a different system apply depending on where the incident took place, and not only do different restrictions apply depending on the circumstances, but each procedure is entirely different and governed by its own rules or, in the absence of rules, by its own ethos.

4.2.1 NHS hospitals

The first point to be made about the hospital complaints procedure is that it does not apply to hospitals outside the NHS. How anyone can justify a situation where if treatment takes place in a private hospital there is no recognized procedure for complaining is difficult to comprehend.

There are two possibilities. Firstly it may simply be the crudest operation of the market ethic: if someone is prepared to pay for a service then they should let the market handle complaints; alternatively it may have been that because the private sector was so small the government did not think that it was worthwhile to tackle the very real difficulties which would present themselves in trying to deal with the private sector.

It is to be hoped that neither of these arguments would now be accepted, particularly the latter bearing in mind the growth of the private sector that is being encouraged. Sadly the remit of the Review of Complaints procedures set up in June 1993 (the Wilson Committee) did not extend to the private sector save insofar as a complaint is connected with treatment under the NHS [5].

The basis of the hospital complaints procedure is an internal enquiry triggered by a patient's complaint. The procedure was originally set out in Health Circular (81)5 and subsequently consolidated in Health Circular (88)37 [6]. It comprises three stages.

- The patient complains, initially either verbally to any member of staff but ultimately in writing to the officer who is designated to deal with complaints.

- If the patient is not satisfied with the response the complaint is renewed and it is then considered by or on behalf of the Regional Medical Officer.

- If the Regional Medical Officer considers it appropriate then an Independent Professional Review (IPR) will be arranged whereby two consultants from outside the Region will be asked to investigate the complaint and then see the complainant in consultation to explain their findings.

It is the experience of Action for Victims of Medical Accidents (AVMA) that the vast majority of patients find this procedure unsatisfactory.

The reasons for this are difficult to ascertain because they are inherent in the procedure. Basically it is a secret procedure as far as the patients are concerned. The patients have no input whatsoever. They do not know what investigations are made, do not see the statements made by other parties (and certainly cannot challenge them) and do not have an opportunity to look at their own medical records.

Furthermore the outcome of the enquiry is bound to be one that finds no real fault on the part of the hospital or staff. That is because Health Circular (81)5 provides that *if there is any possibility* [my italics] of litigation then the IPR is not appropriate. In other words it is decided in advance that only the complaints that will have an outcome favourable to or only mildly critical of the institution or its staff can be dealt with by an IPR.

Because of the somewhat loose nature of this procedure an important aspect such as the time limit for making such a complaint is by no means clear. Obviously patients are encouraged to make the complaint timeously but it is generally believed that any complaint brought within twelve months will be dealt with. However adult patients must be careful that delays in the complaints procedure do not mean that they miss the almost inflexible time limits for starting an action if they ultimately wish to bring the matter to court.

4.2.2 *General practitioners*

The procedure for dealing with complaints against GPs could not be more different. This is because it is not a system aimed at dealing with dissatisfied patients but with the relationship of employer and employee, that is, between the doctor and the FHSA. On a complaint being made, the object of the FHSA is simply to ascertain whether there has been a breach of the practitioner's terms of service.

The effect of this is firstly to ensure that the procedure is shackled by over-bureaucratic legalistic procedures and secondly that patients are totally misled into believing that their grievances are going to be addressed. To meet this objection informal conciliation has been developed by many FHSAs and, whilst there are dangers in this for patients, a number of FHSAs have made that procedure work well in the interests of both patients and doctors. This is often because of the personality and skill of the particular conciliator.

The major danger inherent in the conciliation process is that the patient may become involved in it without knowing the facts. Unless the patient is first informed of what really happened and why, the conciliation process may simply lead to the patient accepting a situation which is not a true one and agreeing not to pursue the matter on a false premise. That can not only lead to problems for the patient at a later stage but will also mean that the doctor's behaviour, which may need attention, is never addressed and future patients may suffer in a similar way.

When a patient complains to the FHSA, the Chairperson of the Medical Services Committee, Dental Services Committee or Pharmaceutical Services Committee, as the case may be, will decide whether the complaint warrants a hearing. If so it will be referred for hearing before the appropriate committee. The tribunal comprises a lay chairperson, two other lay members and two GPs. The proceedings before the committee are formal with the patient presenting the case and calling any witnesses, all of whom are subject to cross-examination, followed by a similar procedure for the practitioner.

Neither party can be represented by a professional advocate but the practitioner is usually represented by someone from their defence organization and the patient is often represented by someone from the Community Health Council.

The time limit for complaining is very strict as the complaint must be made to the FHSA within 13 weeks of the incident complained of. This very often works great hardship for the patient as it can frequently be long after 13 weeks before the patient is either well enough to do anything about the incident or indeed realizes that something has gone wrong and there is cause for complaint.

4.2.3 *Problems for the patients*

Although the procedures for the hospital and GPs are totally different, the fundamental problems for the patient are surprisingly similar.

(1) **Delay**. In both cases the enquiry can take many months and sometimes years.

(2) **Inadequate assistance and information**. Whilst the patient can seek help from the Community Health Council, and frequently does, that is often not sufficient to ease the way in a system which appears designed to discourage complaints.

(3) **Lack of independence**. Those involved in the health service frequently maintain that the procedures are adequate because a number of patients are satisfied with the outcome. The flaw in this conclusion is that invariably the satisfied patient is the one who 'succeeds'. The patient whose complaint is not upheld will always believe that the system has beaten them and that the health care professionals have closed ranks against them.

There is enough evidence to suggest that on occasions this does happen. One only has to look at a few litigation cases to find it. The hospital, the doctors concerned and the nurses combine to try and defeat the patient's claim and only after the closest and most persistent investigation does the truth emerge and the defendants often admit, albeit at the door of the court, that mistakes had been made.

Because this is known to happen the patient whose complaint is rejected under the present procedures will remain convinced that an injustice has been done. That is not only damaging to the patient but, in that suspicion and distrust of health carers is fostered, it is damaging to the system of health care itself.

Any system that does not satisfy the twin pillars of natural justice – that justice must be done and must be seen to be done – will not give patients the satisfaction they are seeking.

4.3 The Ombudsman

The proceedings of the Health Service Commissioner, to give the formal title, illustrates this last assertion if such illustration is needed. The Ombudsman can only deal with complaints relating to administrative matters but these can often be as troubling to a patient or relatives as clinical problems.

For example see the Second Report of the Commissioner for Session 1988–89 Case No. W.249/87/88[7]. There the complainant's mother suffered from diverticulitis and was admitted to hospital for treatment. The complaint was that she and her family were led to believe that she was suffering only from diverticulitis whereas a scan carried out prior to her admission to the hospital had shown that she was suffering from a malignant disease and in fact she died shortly after discharge from hospital.

In that type of situation it can be of immense importance for the complainant to find out what exactly happened and to know that those responsible have been brought to account and steps taken to ensure that others do not suffer in a similar way. In the example the finding of the Commissioner was of particular relevance to nurses. He said, *inter alia*:

'I have also noted that members of the nursing staff failed to find out what the complainant's mother knew of her illness and I believe that their failure to complete the initial assessment sheet played some part in this. Although I accept it is not a responsibility of nursing staff to inform a patient of the diagnosis, their failure to discover the extent of the mother's knowledge of her condition and to inform medical staff accordingly merits my criticism.'

The Ombudsman is independent of the Health Service. His enquiries are painstaking and thorough and he has considerable power. The Select Committee on the Health Service has been known to call a consultant before it to give a explanation of matters referred to in the Ombudsman's report and to give him a most uncomfortable time.

There is no formal procedure for complaining to the Ombudsman and any member of the public can write direct. Once the Ombudsman agrees that the issue is one which he is competent to investigate then the matter is left entirely in his hands.

The reports of the Ombudsman which are available to the public give an insight into how different things would be if an independent investigation could take place into all complaints of whatever nature. That is not to suggest that the Ombudsman would be the appropriate person to investigate all complaints including those relating to clinical matters nor that the system is perfect.

The Ombudsman does not have to investigate complex medical issues and a format whereby one person is ultimately responsible for decisions of that kind would leave the postholder vulnerable to the pressures we see operating from the medical establishment in the various other areas where the competence of doctors is challenged.

Furthermore, many of the enquiries can take as long as 18 months to complete. In a conflict between speed and thoroughness the patient will always prefer thoroughness but in matters affecting a clinician's competence and possible injury to a patient a quick investigation is important and it would be essential to have procedures which at least have some hope of achieving speed and thoroughness.

Nevertheless the results of the Ombudsman's enquiries are most encouraging and suggest that the case for an independent system is irresistible.

4.4 Complaints leading to disciplinary proceedings

Disciplinary matters involving doctors are dealt with by the General Medical Council (GMC) while those against nurses are dealt with by the UKCC. The procedures of the two institutions for investigating complaints of misconduct are similar. Both have a committee which investigates complaints to determine whether they should be referred for consideration – called the Preliminary Proceedings Committee.

Both the GMC and the UKCC also have a Professional Conduct Committee which actually hears the complaints. These committees are run on the lines of a court with the Council having to prove the charges of misconduct. The strict rules of evidence apply and both sides, that is to say, the Council and the professional are usually represented by lawyers.

The main difference between the two institutions lies in the definition of the misconduct which is required to trigger a hearing. The UKCC refers to 'conduct unworthy or a nurse, midwife or health visitor'. (Rule 1(2)(k) Nurses, Midwives and Health Visitors (Professional Conduct) Rules 1993 [8]) whilst the GMC refers simply to 'serious professional conduct' (The Medical Act 1983, section 36(1)(b)).

4.5 Case study

4.5.1 The facts

At the age of 82 the complainant's mother suffered a stroke and was hospitalized. The complainant and her siblings were devoted to their mother and were in constant attendance on her while she was in hospital.

She seemed to be making progress and was due to be transferred to a different hospital for rehabilitation. The day before her transfer was due she suffered a set-back and her condition deteriorated. The transfer nevertheless took place. She rallied slightly and the children thought she was improving. So much so that although until then they had been sleeping at the hospital they went home that night. They were called back in the early hours and within a half an hour their mother died.

4.5.2 The complaint

The complainant made a formal complaint to the hospital. Within the constraints of the system the complaint was dealt with in a model manner at least up to the point of the IPR. The Patient Services Manager was courteous and helpful and unusually quick. She furnished the case records, though not obliged to do so, immediately on request.

(Often failure to produce the records is a source of suspicion and dissatisfaction in itself.)

At the conclusion of the review, unlike in so many other cases, she sent a copy of the panel's report to the complainant rather than simply a summary. (Again sending a summary often proves extremely frustrating to a complainant and can often be the main factor which causes a complainant to litigate.) The report was with the complainant by the 27 August 1993 some eight months from the death of her mother.

The complainant was not satisfied and in September 1993 she wrote to AVMA. Her letter finished:

'We had faith in the staff and trusted them with our mother's life. It appears that doctors are playing GOD, and making decisions on who lives and dies. We wanted to care for mother ourselves at home. If she had been incontinent that was no problem she had cared for us when we were and we wanted to care for her. She had worked hard all her life to feed and care for us . . .

We believe the only way we are going to get satisfactory answers is by seeking legal advice and possibly asking an independent medical expert to look at mother's medical records.'

The complainant has now resolved to pursue the matter in the Court.

4.5.3 Discussion

This case study has been selected because it demonstrates that even when the complaint procedure is operated in the best possible way it is not adequate and can result in inappropriate legal proceedings.

What the system failed to do was to satisfy the complainant that the complaint was being investigated from her point of view. What the format of that system suggests to any complainant is that she is fighting the system.

This was reinforced as it often is by the wording used in two particular paragraphs of the letter of explanation sent by the Patient Services Officer.

'While the decision to proceed with the transfer was regrettable, Dr [X] did not feel that your mother's transfer to [Y] Hospital contributed in any way to her further deterioration and subsequent death'; and

'The recurrent chest infections which your mother experienced while in hospital are virtually inevitable following a stroke which causes paralysis of the throat muscles.'

These paragraphs are not an explanation but simply a recording of the very issues which are at stake. A bald statement like that contained in the first paragraph about the very issue which is troubling the complainant, without further explanation and by the very doctor whose treatment is being criticized, can only serve to create suspicion.

Again in the second paragraph there is no explanation as to why and what was done in this case to try and ensure that no infection occurred.

An outside observer can see that a distraught relative will be angered by this response rather than reassured.

The report from the reviewing doctors also provides a clue as to the reason for the complainant's dissatisfaction. The doctors wrote:

'As a result of interviews with various parties involved in the enquiry we felt we were able to answer most questions posed to our own satisfaction. Unhappily many of the answers were not acceptable to the complainants.

It emerged early in the enquiry that behind the many criticisms of management at the [y]hospital were two major concerns. The first was that their mother was put down deliberately by lethal injections of potassium chloride or morphine overdose as a form of euthanasia. The relatives were also critical that antibiotic therapy was withheld in the final days of their mother's illness with the inevitable result of death from chest infection.

From our careful examination of the notes and treatment charts and specific questioning of the doctors and Sister involved, we found no evidence whatsoever to support the accusation that Mrs [Z]'s life had been terminated by potassium chloride or excess morphine dosage.'

They went on:

'Overall our view was that management was conventional and satisfactory. Our only criticism relates to communication to her family of details of Mrs [z]'s final illness and treatment. Some of this communication difficulty may have related to some of the personalities involved. We were concerned by their interpretation of events which was at times unrealistic. Despite trying repeatedly, we were unable to dissuade them that any cover up was operating. Our firm joint opinion expressed was, that there was no evidence of any medical malpractice, but unfortunately we failed to convince the relatives of this.'

It can immediately be seen that the very nature of the complaint was such that the complainant would never be satisfied with a review conducted under the auspices of the offending hospital and with the 'independent' consultants being selected in such a way as to fail to reassure the complainant that they were in fact independent. It was hardly likely that the records or statements taken would have enabled the reviewers to find that the complainant's mother had been 'put down'.

It is more than likely that a truly independent investigation would have arrived at the same conclusion and that the complainant would not have been satisfied. Nevertheless such an investigation would have had a possibility of exposing any unacceptable practice and the complainant would have been aware of this. She might have accepted an unfavourable decision in those circumstances.

What is absolutely essential in all cases, but particularly in a case as potentially controversial as this, is that the investigation must not only be independent but it must be seen to be independent.

On the other hand no purpose is served by using valuable resources in going through a procedure which is bound not to satisfy a complainant.

In a case of this kind the nurse's role could be crucial both in preventing the circumstances which lead to a complaint and in helping the complainant to accept that the investigation has been unbiased.

The complainant had referred in her extremely detailed notes to a number of occurrences which had aroused her suspicions. Indeed, attached to the complaint was a lengthy document containing a detailed record of all the observations made by the family of the mother's treatment throughout her stay in the hospital. For example it was alleged that the doctor at the second hospital had been very helpful until the consultant intervened and then she had avoided her; that a nurse had been observed about to replace a drip only to be pushed aside by the doctor who attached a different bag – the complainant alleged that this bag contained excess potassium chloride which had killed her mother.

If the nurses had explained things to the relatives as events unfolded; if they had, for example, not allowed them to go home at the very point when the patient was about to die; if they had at the time explained why certain treatment was or was not being given, the relatives might not have been so suspicious. Finally if the nurses had acted as advocates on behalf of the relatives once a complaint was being made, as is envisaged by the UKCC advisory document previously referred to in section 4.1, much could have been done to dispel the lack of trust which led to the relatives rejecting the result of the investigation.

4.6   Identifying the need for reform

4.6.1   *The Association of Community Health Councils*

The Association of Community Health Councils for England and Wales (ACHCEW) some years ago identified the necessary ingredients for a satisfactory complaints procedure [9].

(1) **Visibility**. Complaints mechanisms must be publicized.
(2) **Accessibility**. Those with a grievance should be able to lodge it with someone in authority with minimum difficulty.
(3) *Speed*. A speedy resolution to complaints is in the interests of not only the complainant but also those against whom the complaint is made.
(4) **Impartiality**. It is the view of many who have been through them that the existing complaints procedures are beholden to the medical profession.
(5) **Effectiveness**. The outcomes of the different complaints procedures are unclear and often unsatisfactory.

4.6.2 The Patient's Charter

The Patient's Charter recognized some of these needs and in its provisions sets out in a broad-brush manner the principles which could begin to underpin a reasonable system. For example it establishes a new right for patients 'to have any complaint about NHS services – whoever provides them – investigated and to receive a full and prompt written reply from the chief executive or general manager.'

This, coupled with what is recorded as an established right 'to be given a clear explanation of any treatment proposed, including any risks and any alternatives, before you decide whether you will agree to the treatment', establishes in theory a powerful framework of power for patients. As the Charter does not deal with implementation or enforcement of these rights, however, it remains little more than a guideline as to how it is hoped a complaints system will develop.

4.6.3 The Action for Victims of Medical Accidents (AVMA)

AVMA, approaching the problems from a slightly different vantage point in that those consulting them invariably had suffered some damage as a result of the care or lack of it that they had received, nevertheless had vast experience of patients wishing to complain about their treatment. Indeed, the patient invariably wished primarily to receive satisfactory responses to their complaint rather than to deal with the damage suffered.

AVMA came to the same conclusions as ACHCEW as to the requirements for a satisfactory complaints procedure. Because they dealt with accidents, however, it became absolutely clear that any system that attempted to deal solely with complaints and ignored the issue of accidents would not solve the fundamental problem that bedevils the present system of complaints – the need for the patient to believe that the procedure has not been unduly influenced by the health professionals themselves.

What also became clear to both ACHCEW and AVMA, was that, much as the health professionals would like to do so, it was not possible to separate a complaints system from compensation and disciplinary issues. Whilst there are many occasions when a complaint has no other implications, equally there are numerous situations when a patient's complaint may involve both a need for and entitlement to compensation and a necessity for some form of disciplinary action.

The fact that the proliferation of complaints procedures for different types of complaint is unfair to patients (see section 4.2) is now recognized by all those involved in this area. See, for example the evidence to the Wilson Committee (see section 4.8) of such widely different bodies as the British Medical Association (BMA), the Patients Association and the National Association of Health Authorities and Trusts (NAHAT).

It defies logic, therefore, to wish to continue such a complicated system by insisting that complaints *simpliciter* should go to one body, complaints which may attract compensation should go to another and complaints which may involve disciplinary issues should go to a third.

4.7 A health standards inspectorate

To meet these two major problems, that of independence and the need to deal with all the implications of a complaint, ACHCEW and AVMA have jointly published proposals for a health standards inspectorate [9].

It is interesting to note that as an initial reaction, the proposals were, not surprisingly, not well received by the health profession (where it commented at all); the idea of some form of independent inspection has subsequently been suggested by a number of commentators, some of whose interests can be said to lie with that profession itself.

See, for example, the article in *Healthcare Management* November 1993 – 'There is a need for something like OFWAT and OFGAS for the NHS' [10]; the article by Rudolf Klein and Ellie Scrivens in the *Health Service Journal* 25 November 1993 – 'if the purpose is public accountability, then any accreditation system is likely to look remarkably like a national inspectorate' [11]; and a strong letter in that same edition from Rob Yeldham, Director of the NHS Support Federation, in which he argues that 'regional regulatory agencies are required, monitoring and enforcing standards, evaluating efficiency and conducting audits' [12]. He too mentions OFWAT and OFGAS which, he says, 'may have their faults but they are independent of government and the industries that they regulate'.

The fundamental premise of the AVMA/ACHCEW proposals is independence. The inspectorate would be controlled by a board comprising a mixture of lay people and professionals which would be accountable to the Secretary of State for Health. In addition to its reactive role in dealing with complaints, claims and disciplinary matters the inspectorate would also have a proactive role to assist in the maintenance and improvement of standards.

Whilst dealing with complaints properly will always be necessary the objective must be to reduce the cause of complaints as much as is humanly possible. As James Reason, Professor of Psychology at the University of Manchester, explains, forms of recurrent error 'can be moderated by good training, appropriate procedures, well-designed human/machine interfaces and the like, but they can never be entirely eliminated altogether' [13]. However, it is essential that every effort is made to reduce the number of accidents or causes for complaint to an absolute minimum.

The main way of doing that is to improve standards. There are a number of ways of doing that and indeed there are many initiatives in progress at the present time such as clinical audit and risk management programmes.

The disadvantages of both of these are the lack of any patient input and the lack of independence. Whilst there can be no objection to efforts of this kind to improve standards the history of the medical profession suggests that a measure of independence, coupled with a last resort power of coercion and sanctions is an essential element if patient dissatisfaction is to be reduced.

The inspectorate would therefore carry out its role through medically qualified inspectors who would work through the existing procedures where possible.

Under the board (the policy-making and controlling body) there would be four separate commissions to deal with complaints, compensation, discipline and administration. It would not be intended that the existing procedures would be disturbed where they are plainly seen to be working well. For example, other than the time taken, the Ombudsman's process of dealing with administrative matters is well respected by patient and professional alike. The system could be retained in its entirety. Indeed there is scope for extending its methods of investigation and the pool from which it draws its investigators to the inspectorate. The difference would be that the Ombudsman would be within the inspectorate and accountable to the board.

Similarly with the disciplinary procedures of the UKCC, the present structure and the best features could be maintained but again with the board having overall control. Finally the informal procedures for conciliation which are exercised at local level would have to be retained.

The advantage over any of the present systems would be the interrelation between the various commissions. It would no longer be possible for a person successfully to make a complaint but subsequently to find that she or he fails on a claim for compensation because the format of the tribunal or the availability of the evidence has changed. It would also no longer be possible for a finding of gross negligence by a nurse or doctor to be made in one forum but for that person to continue in practice with nobody looking at the question of their fitness to practice. Nor would it be possible, as happens now, for a nurse to be struck off for her part in an incident whjlst the more culpable doctor in the same incident is warned or not even disciplined.

Each separate commission would be entitled, and in certain circumstances required, to pass on to the other appropriate commissions information about any person dealt with in its forum. In addition the inspector concerned would be involved at every stage of the proceedings. Professor Margaret Stacy, writing in the *AVMA Medical and Legal Journal* (Summer 1993)[14] commended the proposals:

> 'Such radical ideas loosen the mind in areas where much is atrophied and it is easy to give up the effort of trying to work out how the job might be better done. Not designed as an attack on healthcare workers, medical or other, the proposals try to work out a radically new system to ensure that the public is properly protected.'

Unfortunately the government, whilst recognizing the totally unsatisfactory nature of the complaints system, has failed to recognize the essential interrelation between complaints, compensation and disciplinary issues. In setting up a committee to look into the present system of complaints and make proposals for change (the Wilson Committee) it had missed a golden opportunity to review comprehensively all the problems facing patients in this area.

4.8 The Wilson Committee Report

In May 1994 the Wilson Committee issued its report for consultation[5]. Although it showed all the signs of the time pressures placed on the committee by the Secretary of State it is a commendable effort to resolve what is a complex issue. The main attributes of the proposals are:

- that it creates one system to deal with all complaints,
- that initially all less complex complaints will be dealt with as near to the source of complaint as possible.
- that those dealing with complaints should be thoroughly trained, and
- that the approach to complaints will be from the complainant's point of view.

Where the report falls down from the patient's point of view is in connection with stage two of the procedure which will deal with the more complex issues and those which have not been resolved at stage one. Here the committee has failed to provide for a hearing which is what patients want above all, and it has left it to the Secretary of State to decide the fundamental issue as to the ownership of the procedure. If the Secretary of State does not opt for a truly independent procedure but leaves the NHS in control then the whole of the proposals will be undermined in the eyes of patients.

Subject to the major reservations expressed, the implementation of the report should lead to a great improvement in the situation relating to complaints. Unfortunately, the failure to link and deal with the other issues previously referred to will undoubtedly mean that the problems for patients and their dissatisfaction with the system will continue. That will be unfortunate for patient-professional relationships and, as a result, for patients and the professionals themselves.

4.9 Notes and references

1. For a discussion of the Davies Committee report see Association of Community Health Councils for England and Wales, *Health News Briefing* 'National Health Service Complaints Procedures: A Review,' London: ACHCEW, 1990 pp 24–7.
2. UKCC *The Code of Professional Conduct for the Nurse, Midwife and Health Visitor*, 3rd edn. London: UKCC, 1992.
3. UKCC *Exercising Accountability*, London: UKCC, 1989.
4. DHSS, *Health Service Complaints Procedure*, HC (81)5, London: DHSS, 1981.
5. The Wilson Committee reported in 1994, Department of Health *Being Heard: The report of a review committee on NHS complaints procedures*, London: DoH, 1994: paras 5 and 6.
6. DHSS, *Hospital Complaints Procedure Act 1985*, HC (88)37, London: DoH, 1981.
7. House of Commons Health Service Commissioner Second Report for Session 1988–89 (House of Commons Paper 343) London: HMSO.
8. The Nurses, Midwives and Health Visitors (Professional Conduct) Rules 1993 Approval Order 1993; S.I. 1993 No. 893 London: HMSO, 1993.
9. ACHCEW, *Health News Briefing*, 'National Health Service Complaints Procedures: A Review, ACHCEW, London, 1990.
10. Caines, E. 'We should boldly go forward'. *Healthcare Management* November 1993 p 7.
11. Klein, R. & Scrivens, N. 'The Bottom Line'. *Health Service Journal* 1993, 25 November, p 26.
12. Yeldham, R. 'We need a watchdog on Trusts' (Letter). *Health Service Journal* 1993, 25 November, p 20.
13. Reason, J.T. 'The Human Factor in Medical Accidents', In: Vincent, C., Ennis, M. & Audley R.J. (eds.), *Medical Accidents*, Oxford; Oxford Medical Publications, 1993.

14. Stacy, M. 'Self-Regulation or Public Regulation.' *The AVMA Medical and Legal Journal* 1993; Vol. 4; No. 3; pp 1–3.

Part Two
The Perspectives

Chapter 5
Negligence

A   The Legal Perspective
Jonathan Montgomery

The law of negligence, also known in the health care context as mal-practice law, is part of what is known as 'tort' law. The term is derived from the old law-French word meaning 'wrong' and this branch of the law deals with injuries caused by one person to another. The doctrine of negligence applies to all areas of human activity, but its operation in relation to health care has some special features. This chapter explains the nature and functions of the negligence law, illustrating it with examples.

Nurses, midwives and health visitors are likely to become involved in malpractice litigation after one of their patients or clients has suffered a serious accident. If such patients need money, to compensate for their inability to work or to pay for help or equipment that they now need, they may decide to sue some of those who cared for them. They would allege that the professionals were responsible for their injuries and should pay the costs that these cause.

The circumstances in which a negligence action may arise are very varied. Any bad mistake might constitute negligence, and it is impossible to illustrate all aspects of this area of law with a single case study. Errors might occur in relation to diagnosis, selecting, delivering or monitoring care (including the administration of medicines), counselling, liaising with other professionals, or checking equipment. This chapter seeks to outline the basic shape of negligence law and to illustrate its application as the legal problems are discussed.

5.1   The functions of negligence law

Tort law is one of the ways in which nurses, midwives and health visitors are held accountable. It differs from other types of law in a number of ways. **Criminal law** establishes standards on behalf of society, and when the rules are broken society punishes the wrongdoer irrespective of the victim's position. The wrong is committed against society as a whole. **Tort law** is concerned with the relationship between individuals.

When mishaps occur, victims can choose whether they wish to sue the person who caused the action. If they decide to sue, and win their case, they will receive compensation, which is designed so far as possible to put them in the position in which they would have been if nothing had happened to them. The major function of negligence actions therefore, in health care as elsewhere, is to provide compensation for the victims of accidents.

The second main function of negligence actions is to provide an incentive to practitioners to attain a high standard of care. The fact that falling short of the proper standards of care may lead to being sued and paying out money is thought to deter poor practice. It must be emphasized, however, that this function of tort law is very different from the role of the UKCC in maintaining and raising standards. The UKCC is interested in ensuring that the highest standards are attained. The law of negligence is concerned to guarantee that a minimal level of competence is achieved. The standard of care in negligence does not represent the quality of care that nurses, midwives and health visitors should aspire to provide, it establishes the basic standard of practice that patients are entitled to expect as a minimum.

5.2 Negligence law in outline

To win a negligence case against a nurse, midwife or health visitor, a patient/client needs to prove three things. If the court is not satisfied that they have all been proved, then the case will fail. The first is whether the professional sued was responsible for the victim's care at the time of the mishap (i.e. whether they had a 'duty of care' towards them). The second issue concerns the standard of care given. The person suing (the 'plaintiff') has to show that the person being sued (the 'defendant') failed to act in a manner acceptable to their professional peers. Finally, victims have to show that the injuries that they suffered were caused by the failure to practise properly, and not by some independent accident.

Each of these three questions:

- 'Was the professional responsible for the patient?'
- 'Did she fail in her responsibility?'
- 'Did her failure injure the patient?'

raises its own legal complexities. However, the essence of a negligence case lies in answering them.

5.3 The duty of care

5.3.1 *The extent of the duty*

In many cases, it is obvious that a nurse, midwife or health visitor owes someone a duty of care. Where patients are in hospital, the ward staff are clearly responsible for their care. Sometimes, however, things are more difficult. Are nurses responsible for the well-being of their patients' relatives? Are they obliged to assist the victims of accidents? Are they liable for injuries to their colleagues?

The legal test for the extent of duties of care in negligence is designed to answer this sort of question.

5.3.2 The link with the victim

The first step is to consider whether it is reasonably foreseeable that the victim could be affected by the defendant's actions. If the nurse, midwife or health visitor could have foreseen that what she did would affect another person, than she should have borne that person's interests in mind. That does not mean that she is always bound to do what is best for everyone whom she knows she will affect. The question of how she should consider their interests is an aspect of the 'standard of care' issue.

That first stage in answering the duty of care question is likely to result in a long list of people whose position might be altered by a practitioner's actions. This list can sometimes be shortened. The first way to do this is to argue that the connection between the victim and the defendant is too remote for the law to be interested in it. If the connection between the nurse, midwife and health visitor and the victim is very tenuous, then the courts might accept that it is inappropriate to hold the professional responsible.

The principal example of this type of limitation is the fact that there is no legal obligation to help the victims of an accident merely because they might benefit from assistance. In general, a nurse, midwife or health visitor who passes a road traffic accident has no obligation to stop and minister to anybody who has been injured.

The only circumstances in which she would have a duty of care towards that person, and would therefore be bound to help, are when she is already under such a duty because of her job. Thus, a district nurse or health visitor employed to give care to anybody who presents needing it in a geographical area might be obliged by her contract of employment to stop and care for an accident victim. A community midwife who became aware that one of her women was in difficulties would need to offer assistance because she has a general obligation to provide the necessary support.

5.3.3 Restriction as a matter of public policy

The second way to limit the scope of the duty of care is to appeal to arguments of public policy. A duty of care will only exist when it is 'just and reasonable'. Where widening the obligations of health professionals would adversely affect patient care (see sections 5.7.2 and 5.7.3), it is probable that the courts would shy away from such an extension. Examples, from the health care context, of the second type of limitation are difficult to find in the judgments of the courts. However, in the Congenital Disabilities (Civil Liability) Act 1976, parliament has imposed an important restriction on actions in relation to unborn children which has the effect of limiting duties of care. Under the Act, children may sue in respect of injuries suffered before they were born, but only if a duty of care owed to their mothers has been broken. The implication of this rule is that, in law, midwives are not faced with a conflict of duties between the child and mother. Their legal duty is to the mother. If they fail to carry out that duty properly they may be liable to both the mother and to the child. But they cannot be liable for pre-natal injuries to the child if they have cared properly for the mother.

5.3.4 *Duty to non-patients/clients*

In the light of these principles, it can be seen that there will rarely be circumstances when a nurse, midwife or health visitor owes a legal duty of care to a stranger who is the victim of an accident (although she may feel under a moral obligation). It should be noted, however, that even though the law would not impose a duty of care in these circumstances, a professional who stops to help will be taken to have freely chosen to accept such a duty. This means that they may not simply give up caring for the victim. Further, their help must be reasonably competent, because the standard of care (see section 5.4) must be satisfied.

In relation to the other categories of people to whom a duty of care might exist, it will often be wholly foreseeable that a relative will be directly affected by a health professional's actions. For example, if an infectious patient were to be carelessly discharged from hospital it would be foreseeable that they might infect others, so that proper precautions would be necessary. Careless acts at work will obviously put colleagues at risk, and therefore a duty of care to them would exist.

The crucial point, however, is that the fact that a duty of care exists is only the first step. Failure to reach the required standard of care must also be proved. This standard will often be quite low in relation to people other than the patient/client because it will normally be quite proper to put the patient's interests first.

5.4 Breach of the standard of care

5.4.1 *The Bolam test*

The standard of care required of health professionals was established in a case in 1957 called *Bolam* v. *Friern Hospital Management Committee*. That case held that 'a doctor is not guilty of negligence if he has acted in accordance with a practice accepted as proper by a responsible body of medical men [sic] skilled in that particular art.'

This test has been adopted by the House of Lords in a number of cases and is now applied to all health professionals.

The essence of the *Bolam* test is that professionals are to be judged against the standards of their peers. Nurses midwives or health visitors will successfully defend themselves against a negligence action if the experts from their profession who are called to give evidence are prepared to accept that their actions were proper. That does not mean that the experts would have done the same, but they regard the defendant's actions as within the range of acceptable practice. It is important to note that they are looking for the minimal level of acceptable practice, not what they would like to have seen happen.

In many cases there will be disagreements amongst professionals about how problems should be handled. The House of Lords has explicitly said that it will not choose between different schools of medical opinion. They went on to say that fitting in with one acceptable school of thought is a sufficient defence to a negligence claim, even though another body of professional opinion might be vehemently opposed to it (*Maynard v. West Midlands Regional Health Authority* (1985)).

It is not clear whether the same lenience would be shown to nurses, midwives and health visitors as is shown to doctors. The courts are extremely reluctant to challenge medical clinical judgment, possibly because they feel unable to comprehend medical practice [1]. They may feel that the expertise of nurses, midwives and health visitors is less esoteric, and be less wary of judging it.

As well as recognizing that there is room for disagreement amongst responsible professionals, the courts have accepted that nurses, midwives and health visitors do not work in a vacuum. A number of issues are raised. How far does experience matter? Would following instructions provide a defence to an accusation of negligence? What is the significance of hospital policies? Can there be liability for mistakes made by a colleague?

5.4.2 *Trainees and supervision*

It is clear that the law imposes the same standard of care on students as on trained staff. This is a general principle, established in *Nettleship* v. *Weston* (1971), a case that held that a learner driver would be liable in negligence if he failed to drive as well as a reasonably competent qualified driver. This may seem harsh, but the justification for the rule is that patients/clients are entitled to expect that they will receive a proper standard of care.

Students must learn how to practise properly, but it would not be fair to impose the burden of their training on their patients. At the same time, the real fault may lie with qualified staff who have failed to provide proper support and guidance for the students. Such a failure may itself be negligent, and may enable the student to claim reimbursement from their employer should she have to pay damages to a patient (*Jones* v. *Manchester Corporation* (1952).

However, subject to the rule about learners, the standard of care is partly tailored to the position a nurse, midwife or health visitor holds in the health care team. A sister would be judged against the standards to be expected of all reasonable sisters. A specialist nurse would be judged against the proper practice of specialists in her field.

It is also important to note that there is more than one way for a junior member of staff to meet their obligations. The law recognises, as does the UKCC Code of Conduct, that practitioners should recognise their limitations. Where a professional is unsure that they can provide the necessary care, they may call for assistance. If a mistake is made, but a more experienced person has been called in to check it, then the very calling for help is a responsible thing to do and will usually provide a defence (*Wilsher* v. *Essex Area Health Authority* (1986)). In some cases, it will be appropriate to seek the assistance of a more experienced member of the same profession. In others, referral to a practitioner of a different sort, such as a midwife calling in an obstetrician, would be in order. Failing to summon appropriate help when all responsible practitioners would do so would in itself be negligent on the *Bolam* test.

5.4.3 *Obeying instructions*

Instances where senior practitioners are involved provide examples of a cases where nurses, midwives or health visitors might be faced with a dilemma because they have received instructions that they are unhappy about. Could they be accused of negligence if they followed mistaken advice? It is certainly true that professionals remain personally responsible for their practice, even when they seek advice from others. However, the Court of Appeal has recognized that following the instructions of a doctor will usually provide a nurse with a defence to negligence, even if the directions turn out to be improper (*Gold* v. *Essex County Council* (1942)) [2].

However, in the same case, it was said that a nurse should challenge a prescription that appears improper:

'If a doctor in a moment of carelessness ... ordered a dose which to an experienced ward sister was obviously incorrect and dangerous ... it might well be negligence if she administered it without obtaining confirmation from the doctor or higher authority.'

It would seem from this that if confirmation was forthcoming, the nurse would be protected even if the dose turned out to be wrong. However, the case is over 50 years old and nowadays to be safe it might be wise to follow the UKCC's advice [3] and demand that the doctor administer the drugs.

The last example concerned inter-professional conflict. The expertise of doctors is different from that of nurses, midwives or health visitors. It is right to distribute responsibility for the various tasks of care to the appropriate professions, and to recognize that distribution by permitting practitioners to rely on their colleagues' skill. The position may be slightly different when the instructions come from a more senior member of the same profession because the junior practitioner can be expected to be able to recognize gross errors.

In a case involving two doctors, one junior and the other a consultant, the House of Lords suggested that if instructions were 'manifestly wrong' it would be negligent to carry them out. The consultant had ordered treatment for a fractured arm, but had not mentioned penicillin. The junior doctor was sued for failing to prescribe the drug. She defended herself by arguing that she was properly following the instructions she had been given. It was found that the instructions were not 'manifestly wrong' but merely 'unsuitable and improper' and that the junior doctor was therefore not negligent in deferring to the consultant's expertise (*Junor* v *McNicol* (1959)) There is probably, therefore, a stronger legal duty to question the views of colleagues from the same profession than there is to challenge the expertise of someone from a different profession altogether.

Sometimes, general instructions on the way in which nurses, midwives and health visitors should practice are issued by employers in the form of hospital policies. As employees professionals are obliged to follow lawful and reasonable instructions and may be dismissed for not doing so. This clearly provides an incentive to follow policies. So does the law of negligence, because a failure to follow an established protocol may be evidence of negligence. In one case, a nurse working in a well-woman clinic failed to refer a woman complaining of a lump in her breast to a doctor, as the protocol indicated. She was held to be negligent (*Sutton* v. *Population Family Planning Programme Ltd* (1981)). However, this does not mean that every departure from a hospital policy would be negligent, Where nurses, midwives or health visitors have good clinical reasons for treating a particular client differently this would be accepted by the courts provided a responsible body of professional opinion would support their actions. [4]

5.4.4 *Mistakes of others and vicarious liability*

Next, it is necessary to consider whether professionals might be responsible for mistakes made by others. This is particularly important in relation to the system of primary nursing where a named practitioner is given overall responsibility for a patient's care. Is she therefore liable whenever a mistake is made, irrespective of who made it? The answer to this question is 'no'. Liability for the negligence of someone else can only arise through the doctrine of vicarious liability. This applies to the employer/employee relationship, so that a health authority would be liable for the negligence of those who work for it, but it does not cover the relationship with colleagues or subordinates.

Nevertheless, the person with overall responsibility must exercise that role properly. Some mistakes may at first seem to be the fault of the person carrying out the immediate care but on closer scrutiny may be the result of a failure to give clear instructions or to communicate information about the patient properly. A named nurse or midwife who has charge of a person's care must co-ordinate that care properly, and if she does so negligently will be liable for any damage that results. It is important to note, however, that the practitioner is being held responsible for her own actions here, not for those of other members of the team.

5.5 Proving that damage was caused by negligent behaviour

5.5.1 Damage caused by other factors

The third step in winning a negligence action is proving that the victim suffered damage as a result of the defendant's poor conduct. It does not matter, for the purposes of negligence law, how badly a nurse, midwife of health visitor practices if no injury is suffered. In one case, a patient was sent away from casualty, complaining of stomach pain, without a proper examination and told to see his GP if the symptoms persisted. Before he could do this he had died. The doctor, who had refused to see the man, had clearly failed to act responsibly and in that sense was negligent. However, the evidence showed that even if the man had been examined and the problem correctly diagnosed he would still have died. He had been suffering from arsenic poisoning and it would have been too late to administer an antidote (*Barnett* v. *Chelsea and Kensington Hospital Management Committee* (1968)). This meant that the unacceptable conduct of the doctor made no difference. Even if he had acted properly, the man would still have died. Consequently the claim against the doctor failed because it had not been proved that the injury to the man had been caused by he defendant's conduct.

5.5.2 Problems of proof

In many cases, proving that injury has been caused by the defendant is very difficult. Any uncertainty will operate in favour of the defendant. A patient's legal action will fail unless it can be shown that it was more probable that the injuries were caused by professional negligence than by some other innocent cause. Often it cannot be proved that the patient's injuries were not the result of natural causes; either by their underlying medical problems or by an unavoidable accident. In one case involving a prematurely born child it was possible that the blindness suffered by the child was a consequence of being born at an early stage of development rather than the result of his poor care, even though that had been negligent. Unless it could be proved that the poor care, and not the prematurity, probably caused the blindness, the child could not win the case (*Wilsher* v. *Essex Area Health Authority* (1988)).

An important rule has been established in cases of misdiagnosis. The courts will not recognize the loss of a chance of recovery as enough to prove that injury has been caused by a mistake (*Hotson* v. *East Berkshire Area Health Authority* (1987)). It is not enough to show that, if a proper diagnosis had been made, treatment could have been offered that would have given the patient a chance of recovery. It must be shown that the treatment would probably have worked.

It is, therefore, clear that negligent conduct which does not cause injury will not result in legal liability. This shows that the primary function of negligence law is as a means of compensating the victims of accidents, not to ensure high standards. Practitioners cannot know in advance whether damage might result leading to causation being proved. They can only assess whether their actions would receive the support of their peers, and thus satisfy the legal standard of care. They should therefore concentrate on practising well and not worry about the legal technicalities of causation.

5.6 The calculation of damages

If plaintiffs win their cases, they are entitled to 'damages', an amount of money to compensate them for their injuries. General principles apply when calculating them, no special rules exist for medical accident cases [5]. Under these rules, damages are made up of a number of categories.

5.6.1 Compensation for injuries – 'general' damages

First, there is 'fair and reasonable' compensation for the injury suffered. This is inevitably somewhat arbitrary, as there can be no precise determination of the value of a limb or organ, and the courts have developed an approximate tariff in order to achieve consistency (and this has been formalized by guidelines published by the Judicial Studies Board [6]). Damages will also include a figure for the pain and suffering and loss of amenity experienced by the victim.

5.6.2   *Expenses, loss of earnings and cost of future care – 'special' damages*

These first two categories of damages cannot be calculated precisely, but other losses can be proved more reliably and can then be recovered by the plaintiff. Expenses incurred as a result of the injuries up until the court hearing can be claimed. So can loss of earnings up to that point. The court then needs to speculate as to future losses that will flow from the injuries. It has to estimate the difference between the money that the patient would have earned if the accident had not happened and that which will be earned in the light of any disability suffered. This involves both calculating the annual sum and working out the patient's life expectancy, so that the money lost over the whole lifetime can be recompensed. In essence, this suggests multiplying the estimated annual loss of earnings by the number of years the patient is expected to live. In practice, however, the courts will only multiply the figure by 18, even when the patient is expected to live longer. Payment is also made to provide for adaptions, if required, to the patient's home and the cost of future care. In the case of, for example, a brain damaged child this can be a very large sum.

5.6.3   *Actual loss not 'exemplary' damages*

The important point to note about the process of calculating damages, is that the courts are trying to assess what the patient has lost and will lose. Damages reflect real costs, not punishment for the defendant. Sometimes the sums awarded in damages are vast, over £1 million, but they will only be so large when the patient can show that they have really lost out, and will continue to do so in the future, to that extent as a result of the accident. The mere fact that the payment made is very big does not make it excessive if the injuries and resulting losses are also extensive. There are circumstances when awards include an extra element to reflect the fact that a defendant's wrongdoing was particularly heinous (exemplary damages), but it is hard to envisage them arising in the context of health care [7].

5.7   Negligence law in practice

The bulk of this chapter so far has been concerned to examine the legal principles of negligence. However it is also important to consider the operation of the law in practice. Three areas will be considered. First, who actually gets sued? Second, is there some sort of malpractice crisis in the UK such as is alleged to exist in the United States of America? Third, how should practitioners respond to malpractice law – should they practise so called 'defensive medicine'?

5.7.1 *Who gets sued?*

Although every nurse, midwife and health visitor is personally accountable for the quality of her practice through the law of negligence, it is rare for an individual practitioner to be sued. Cases are fought in order to obtain compensation, and individuals can rarely be guaranteed to have the financial resources to pay damages. In practice, it is usually the professional's employer who is sued. The plaintiff can be confident that they will have the resources to meet a successful claim.

This is possible for two reasons. First, because employers are liable for any negligent acts committed by their employees under the doctrine of 'vicarious liability'. This does not absolve the employee of liability, and patients could choose to sue an individual. However, they may also elect to bring their legal action against the hospital, NHS Trust or health authority for whom the professional worked. They may not receive damages twice over, but it does not matter whether they go to the employee or employer first. In theory and subject to any terms in the employment contract, the employer could seek reimbursement from the negligent employee for anything they had to pay out. However, in practice, this is rarely, if ever, done.

The second way in which the employers could made be liable is through the principle of direct liability [8]. This approach makes provider organizations liable for operating properly the services that they offer to their patients/clients. Legal liability arises out of the organization's promise to provide services. If they fail to do so through negligence, then they must compensate anybody who suffers injury as a result. If the organization promises to deliver a service and fails to do so, it does not matter whose fault it is, the organization as a whole is at fault.

Whichever of these two routes is used to make employers liable, the nurse, midwife or health visitor is likely to be involved in the case. The court would have to be satisfied that the appropriate standard of care had not been given, and it is unlikely that this could be established without involving the practitioners caring for the patient. It might, therefore, feel as though the practitioner was being sued, but it would not be her money that was on the line. Health professionals often feel that their reputation is at stake in malpractice cases. Lawyers tend to see the matter differently. They usually believe that momentary lapses are inevitable and do not reflect on the general standards of competence of the practitioner. On this view, being sued is nothing to be ashamed of unless it constitutes a pattern.

Within the NHS, there is an established procedure [9] that ensures that NHS Trusts or health authorities (whichever employs the practitioner) administer and settle claims. Strictly speaking the arrangements apply specifically to doctors and dentists. However, the same procedure would be followed in respect of cases against nurses midwives and health visitors. This protects professionals from the financial consequences of malpractice litigation. However, it can also lead to health authorities and trusts deciding to settle claims out of court, even when they might be won, because it sometimes makes commercial sense to save on legal costs and avoid the risk of losing.

5.7.2   Is there a malpractice crisis?

There is considerable discussion [10] in the health care press of a supposed malpractice crisis. Litigation is presented as a major threat to health care practice, forcing health care professionals to alter their practice to the detriment of patients and even to give up their work completely. In fact the evidence [11] is complex. It is certainly true that more cases are being started, and that more money is being paid out in damages. However, it is far from clear whether more cases are being won by patients.

In fact, it is far more difficult to win a malpractice action against a health professional than it is to sue for other types of personal injury. A smaller proportion of medical cases are won by plaintiffs than is usual [12]. The standard of care is defined in a more generous way for health professionals than others [13]. Causation is often difficult to prove, and uncertainty protects the health professionals. Insurance is generally cheaper for health professionals than for the members of other professions [14], and in any event does not strictly need to be carried in respect of NHS work [15]. It is difficult to accept that there is a crisis for individual practitioners.

However, it is probably true that malpractice litigation presents a significant problem for the NHS. An increasing amount of money is being paid out in damages and legal costs. Any funds used for this purpose have to be taken from the pool of resources available for patient care. On the other hand, to deny patients injured through negligence any compensation would be unjust. It would leave the patients, who are wholly innocent victims, to bear the financial burdens of their injuries. For a case to be won, it must be shown that the health service was at fault, and it is only just that they rather than the innocent victim should pay.

5.7.3   Defensive practice

Probably the most significant claim made about a possible malpractice crisis concerns the phenomenon of defensive practice. The precise meaning of this term is a matter for debate. However, the essence of the concept is that health professionals are obliged to practise in a way that they believe is bad for their patients/clients because they are trying to avoid being sued. It is claimed that unnecessary tests are performed, and that patients are denied operations that are thought to be risky even though they seem to be best for them.

Hard evidence of the existence of defensive practices is, in fact, difficult to find [16]. Where it does happen, it is based on a misunderstanding of the law. Under the *Bolam* test (discussed in section 5.4.1), the standard of care required by the law is primarily a professional standard, and only a legal requirement because it is a professional one. It follows that the only effective defensive practice is responsible professional practice. There is no point in worrying about the law of negligence. If practitioners ensure that their peers would regard their practice as proper, they will also be ensuring that they have not been negligent.

5.7.4 Conclusion

The law of negligence is an important legal mechanism for holding nurses, midwives and health visitors accountable. Clearly professionals need to be aware of its requirements. They also need to be aware of its wider implications for health services. However, it would be wrong to regard malpractice law as a threat to good practice. The law reinforces professional standards, it does not undermine them. All that the law of negligence requires is that professionals act responsibly according to their own standards of conduct.

5.8 Notes and references

1. See Montgomery, J. 'Medicine, accountability and professionalism.' *Journal of Law and Society* 1989: Vol. 16: pp 319–39.
2. see further, Montgomery, J., 'Doctors' handmaidens: the legal contribution.' In: Wheeler, S., McVeigh, S., eds., *Law health and medical regulation*. Aldershot: Dartmouth 1992, pp 155–7.
3. UKCC, *Exercising Accountability*, London: UKCC, CL.G4. 1989.
4. see further Montgomery, J., 'Doctors handmaidens: the legal contribution.' In: Wheeler, S., McVeigh S., eds., Law health and medical regulation. Aldershot: Dartmouth, 1992, pp 162–3.
5. see Jones, M.A. *Medical Negligence*, London: Sweet and Maxwell, 1991, pp 325–56.
6. for details see Kemp and Kemp *The Quantum of Damages*, London: Sweet and Maxwell, looseleaf, 1993.
7. see Jones, M.A. *Medical Negligence*, London: Sweet and Maxwell, 1991, pp 326–7.
8. Bettle, J., 'Suing hospitals direct: whose tort is it anyhow?' *New Law Journal* 1987; 137; pp 573–7; and Montgomery, J., 'Suing hospitals direct: what tort?' *New Law Journal*, 1987; 137, pp 703–5.

9. Department of Health, *Claims of medical negligence against hospital and community doctors and dentists*, HC (89) 34. 1989.

10. see for example Acheson, Sir D., 'Are obstetrics and midwifery doomed? *Midwives Chronicle*, 1991; pp 158–66.

11. Quam, L., Dingwall, R., Fenn, P., 'Medical malpractice in perspective.' *British Medical Journal* 1987; Vol. 294, pp 1529–32, 1597–1600; Fenn, P., Whelan, C. 'Medical litigation trends, causes and consequences' in: Dingwall, R., ed. *Socio-legal aspects of medical practice.* London: Royal College of Physicians, 1989; and Fenn, P., Dingwall, R. 'The tort system and information: some comparisons between the UK and the US' In: Dingwall, R., Fenn, P., eds., *Quality and Regulation in Health Care: international perspectives.* London: Routledge, 1992.

12. Pearson, *Report of the Royal Commission on Civil Liability and Compensation for Personal Injury*, Cmnd 7054–I, London: HMSO, 1978 p 284; and Fenn, P., Whelan, C. 'Medical litigation: trends, causes and consequences' In: Dingwall, R., ed. *Socio-Legal aspects of medical practice.* London: Royal College of Physicians, 1989, p 8.

13. Montgomery, J. 'Medicine, accountability and professionalism.' *Journal of Law and Society* 1989; Vol. 16; p 322.

14. Ham, C., Dingwall, R., Fenn, P., Harris, D. *Medical Negligence: Compensation and Accountability*, London: Kings Fund, 1988, pp 13–14.

15. Department of Health, *Claims of medical negligence against hospital and community doctors and dentists*, HC(89) 34. 1989.

16. See Jones, M.A., Morris, A.E. 'Defensive medicine: myths and facts.' *Journal of the Medical Defence Union*, 1989; Vol. 5, pp 40–43.

B An Ethical Perspective – Negligence and Moral Obligations
Graham C. Rumbold and *Harry Lesser*

5.9 The different viewpoints of law and ethics

5.9.1 *The effect of outcome*

The main difference between the legal position on negligence, excellently explained by Mr Montgomery, and an ethical position is that the moral obligations of a carer are normally seen as going beyond the legal obligations, and requiring more to be done. In the first place, for a successful legal action for negligence to be brought, the plaintiff has to be able to prove that they suffered damage or harm as a result of the professional's action or omission (section 5.2). Hence, a professional might, for example, expose a patient to serious and unnecessary risk; but if by good luck no harm followed, there would be no ground for an action for negligence. Clearly, though, the professional would be morally to blame, if the risk were serious and needless. The law bases its judgment on the **actual** effects of actions, whereas ethics, both general and professional, is concerned with the rightness or wrongness of actions themselves, and their **potential** effects. For ethics, negligence is always to be avoided, even if it turns out by good fortune to do no harm.

5.9.2 *What level of care?*

Secondly, the law, by its nature, cannot enforce an ideal standard of care, which would obviously not be practicable. Instead, its aim is to prevent care falling below an acceptable minimum standard: 'The law of negligence is concerned to guarantee that a minimal level of competence is achieved' (section 5.9). Even if this minimum is reasonably high, it inevitably falls short of what professionals have a duty to aim at. Indeed Montgomery continues, 'The standard of care in negligence does not represent the quality of care that nurses, midwives and health visitors should aspire to provide, it establishes the basic standard of practice that patients are entitled to expect as a minimum'.

For, while the law requires professionals only to maintain this basic standard, ethics requires them to do their best not to harm the patient and positively to help them. (There is of course sometimes a problem of knowing what is in the interests of the patient or client; but this is a different issue.) This is brought out in at least three passages in the UKCC *Code of Professional Conduct for the Nurse, Midwife and Health Visitor* of 1992[1].

The first, the second clause of the Code, is a version of what is often called the principle of **non-maleficence**, the principle that nurses, midwives and health visitors, as indeed all health care workers, have a duty not to do harm to patients and clients:

'As a registered nurse, midwife or health visitor . . . you must ensure that no action or omission on your part, or within your sphere of responsibility, is detrimental to the interests, condition or safety of patients and clients.'

The other two passages, in contrast, deal with **beneficence**, with positively helping the patient or client. The Code says

'Each registered nurse, midwife and health visitor shall act, at all times, in such a manner as to promote the interests of individual patients and clients'

and goes on to say

'You must act always in such a manner as to promote and safeguard the interests and well-being of patients and clients.'

This clearly implies a higher expectation than that required by the law of negligence.

There is, though, a problem in deciding what the ethical standard of care should be, and when failure to meet the standard would count as negligence. If it is a minimal standard, as in the law, this fails to take account of the fact that many nurses, whilst operating significantly above the minimal standard, may still believe that they have failed in a way which is blameworthy. On the other hand, we cannot apply the standard of the 'best possible care', which is appropriate only as an ideal to aim at, without stretching the concept of negligence to absurdity.

Perhaps we should distinguish four levels of care. There is, first, the minimum acceptable level, required by the law, which defines legal negligence. There is the higher level required by the Code of Conduct, which defines professional negligence. At the top is 'the best possible care': ethically, health professionals are obliged to **aim** at this (in cases where it is clear what it involves), but are not negligent or blameworthy if they fail to achieve it – ethics is for humans, not angels. In between the second and third of these are the personal standards of individual professionals.

5.10 Problems with ethical standard setting

5.10.1 *Where to set one's standards?*

The problem is whether a person should consider themselves negligent if they meet the requirements of the Code of Conduct but fall short of a possible higher standard – for example, by promoting the well-being of a patient, but not as much as they could. If one says 'no', one risks turning the Code of Conduct into a maximum which no one is prepared to exceed; if one says 'yes', one risks encouraging professionals to adopt impractically high standards, to the detriment of patients and clients as well as themselves. Perhaps this is a matter which individual professionals must decide for themselves.

5.10.2 Balancing risks and harm

There is also another difficulty. To avoid being negligent, one must do one's best both to avoid doing harm and to promote well-being. But most, perhaps all, forms of care, involve some degree of harm or risk, whether in the form of pain and discomfort or in the form of injury and, sometimes, the risk of death. So how are these to be reconciled? What seems to be required here is, first, always (if possible) to consult the patient, so that risks are run and harm endured with their consent and approval; secondly, to avoid unnecessary risks, not required for the sake of a likely benefit; and thirdly, not to inflict harm clearly greater than the benefit to the patient or client. In short, if it is agreed that it is one's duty to do good and avoid doing harm, in so far as these are possible and consistent, one will have to do more than simply meet the standard required by the law, or even the Code of Conduct.

5.10.3 Moral duties

Thirdly, there are occasions when, though there is no legal duty of care, there may well be an ethical duty. Montgomery points out (section 5.3.2) that 'there is no legal obligation to help the victims of an accident merely because they might benefit from assistance.' Hence nurses, midwives or health visitors have no legal obligation to stop and assist victims of accidents, unless they are already under a duty to help the person in question because of their contract of employment. But if we hold that one has an obligation to help those in need, if one can, then they do have a moral obligation. They have at least the same moral duty to help those in need as any other person; and arguably they have a stronger duty than most others, because they have greater relevant knowledge and more skills which will enable them to help the person.

If this is so, then to fail to offer assistance is both morally and professional negligent – professionally, because their particular skills mean they have a special obligation to help, as well as the general obligation we all have. Moreover, once care is offered, it becomes subject to legal as well as moral obligations; it may be judged, particularly if the victim suffers harm as a result of their ministrations, and will be expected to be of a reasonable standard. So it is important that assistance is not half-hearted, and that once involved nurse midwives or health visitors act as if the accident victim were under their professional care.

5.10.4 *Responsibility for the actions of others*

Another area where professional and ethical obligations exist when there are no legal ones concerns 'the system of primary nursing where a named practitioner is given overall responsibility for a patient's care' (section 5.4.4). The named nurse (or other practitioner) is legally responsible for the negligence of other members of the team only if that 'negligence' is the result of her own acts or omissions, for example 'a failure to give clear instructions or to communicate information about the patient properly' or a failure to ensure that those to whom the care has been delegated were adequately informed of their responsibilities and competent to carry them out.

However, clause 2 of the UKCC Code of Conduct (section 5.9.2), by referring to 'your sphere of responsibility', would appear to take this a stage further: it implies that named practitioners remain morally and professionally responsible for the standard of care given by those to whom they delegate the care, and must therefore, in ways consistent with good working relationships, keep a check that standards are maintained.

5.11 Law and ethics in conflict

5.11.1 *The unborn child*

In two other situations – perhaps the most complex we have to deal with – not only is there an ethical duty where there is no legal duty, but also there is the possibility that ethics might require one to act against what is required by the law. The first case concerns unborn children. Montgomery points out (section 5.3.3) that midwives and other health professionals have no legal duty of care to unborn children: 'Their legal duty is to the mother . . . they cannot be liable for pre-natal injuries to the child if they have cared properly for the mother.' Ethically, however, they have a duty to both the mother and the child: the purpose of midwifery and obstetric care is to ensure a safe delivery with the least possible harm occurring to the newborn.

Where the interests of the mother and child are compatible, there is no moral problem: one may say that the legal duty is, until birth, only to the mother, but the ethical duty is to mother and child, so that whatever benefits the child should be done, even if there is no direct benefit to the mother. (Normally, of course, this is in accordance with the mother's wishes, in any case.)

In those rare cases where there is a conflict between the needs of the mother and the child law and ethics divide more sharply. Legally, the duty of the health professional is always to the mother: morally, this is very much a disputed matter, and it may well be that different circumstances require different actions, depending, for example, on the relative risks of possible courses of action and on the mother's own wishes. It is, however, important to note that it is certainly possible, though hopefully very rare in practice, for health professionals to decide that they had an ethical duty to the child which conflicted with their legal duty to the mother.

5.11.2 *To obey instructions or prevent wrong?*

The second case is that of a health professional who is given instructions that they believe to be wrong or mistaken. Montgomery explains (section 5.4.3) that under such circumstances the law requires the orders to be questioned, but does not regard the nurse, for example, as negligent if they are confirmed by the doctor or higher authority before being acted on. (He notes, though, that in such cases 'it might be wise to follow the UKCC's advice and demand that the doctor administer the drugs'.) Moreover he goes on to point out that failure to follow established hospital policy may be evidence of negligence, unless there are 'good clinical reasons for treating a particular client differently'.

Now ethically this may not be enough. For occasionally an established policy, or a particular decision, may be so potentially harmful that it is not enough for the health professional only to question it, or only to demand that the doctor carry it out personally, or even only to exempt a particular client from it – all of which is part of their legal duty. If the consequences, for example, of giving a drug were sufficiently terrible, it would seem that there could be a moral duty not only to refuse to give the drug but also to prevent the doctor from so doing.

The problem is this. Whilst clearly nurses, midwives and health visitors should comply with doctors' orders (if those orders are in the realm of medical practice), nevertheless if in their professional judgment those orders are likely to result in harm to the patient or client they clearly have a moral and professional duty to question them, and even to refuse to carry them out personally: one cannot escape moral responsibility for one's own actions on the basis of obeying orders. As Benjamin and Curtis [2], say

'In so far as a nurse has an obligation to follow a doctor's orders, it is only a prima facie obligation, and may be overridden in certain circumstances by other factors. A nurse must be careful not to confuse a well-grounded prima facie obligation with blind faith.'

Similarly, the UKCC makes it quite clear that each individual nurse, midwife and health visitor is professionally accountable for their own actions.

Again, hospital policy does not remove individual accountability. (Montgomery talks specifically of hospital policy, but the arguments are the same for the employer's policy, for nurses, midwives and health visitors employed by private nursing homes or agencies, GPs or industry). Everything hinges on whether the policy itself accords with agreed professional standards and/or serves the best interests of the patient in question. Whilst it can be argued that one has a moral duty to comply with the policies, rules and regulations of one's employer, this can be justified morally only if the policies, rules and regulations are themselves morally acceptable.

But while the law and the professional code fully support someone who questions an order or policy, and even someone who refuses to carry it out, provided they have good professional grounds, they do not seem to support anyone who actually tries to prevent the order or policy from being executed, or indeed, except in the case of abortion, anyone who has moral objections to a particular policy or procedure of a non-professional kind.

The problem is this. On the one hand, the running of any institution requires that individuals make some sacrifice of their personal judgment of what is best to the judgment of those in charge: life would be impossible if individuals constantly prevented the carrying out of decisions. Moreover, anyone taking this drastic step may well face disciplinary action, and find that, however right they are morally, the law and the Code do not protect them in practice. On the other hand, it can happen that very serious harm will be done if people simply obey orders and take no steps to prevent mistaken or wicked actions.

In the end, each health professional must decide for themselves when the moment has come to put themselves on the line: one hopes most will be spared ever having to make such a decision. The only guideline one might suggest is that normally this should be considered only if the alternative would result in something that would be generally agreed to be seriously harmful, and not in cases where there can be real dispute, such as whether to put the interests of the unborn child above those of its mother. (Even this much is disputable!) But it is important to realize that it can sometimes happen that one's moral duty conflicts with one's legal one and ought to be given precedence over it: exactly when this occurs has to be for the individual to decide.

5.12 Summary

To summarize: a carer has both a legal and an ethical duty to avoid negligence. The ethical duty differs from the legal one in the following ways:

(1) It operates whether or not any harm actually follows from the negligence, since it applies to actions (and failures to act) themselves, and not only to their **actual** consequences, but also to their **potential** ones.

(2) Both with regard to not doing harm and to doing good, the standard of care required by the UKCC Code is higher than that required by the law; and ethics requires that, within reason, a standard higher than both is at least aimed at.

(3) Ethics requires a duty of care towards unborn children, and towards victims of accidents whom one can help, and also a duty to take responsibility for the behaviour of those to whom one has delegated care, which the law does not.

(4) Ethics may occasionally require someone actively to prevent an order or policy from being carried out, even though this may conflict with their legal duty.

5.13 Notes and references

1. UKCC *The Code of Professional Conduct for the Nurse, Midwife and Health Visitor*, London: UKCC 1992.
2. Benjamin, M., Curtis, J. *Ethics in Nursing*, Oxford: Oxford University Press, 1992.

Chapter 6
Consent and The Adult Patient

A The Legal Perspective
Jean McHale

English law requires the nurse [1] to obtain consent from the patient before treatment is given. Without consent a nurse is in danger of being sued for damages in the civil law courts or prosecuted in criminal law. The nurse has two main roles in the consent process. First, when she is acting as the primary carer providing the patient with treatment she has the task of obtaining the patient's consent. The development of the extended role means that the nurse herself will be undertaking this task more often. Second, even if a doctor obtains the patient's consent a patient may be confused or uncertain about her treatment choice and turn to the nurse for advice and clarification.

When complying with her legal obligations in relation to consent to treatment the registered nurse has also to be aware of her professional ethical obligations including her role as advocate for her patient [2]. Here as in other areas of her practice the nurse may find herself torn between what she believes are the obligations required of her under the UKCC professional ethical code and her obligations under her contract of employment.

For the purposes of this chapter I refer to advocacy in the sense that the term is used by the UKCC in their document *Exercising Account-ability* [2]:

'Advocacy is concerned with promoting and safeguarding the well-being and interests of patients and clients. It is not concerned with conflict for its own sake ... Dictionaries define an advocate as "one who pleads the cause of another" or "one who recommends or urges something" and this indicates that advocacy is a positive, constructive activity.'

The advocacy function is still being developed and its boundaries are uncertain.

Consent to treatment is a vast area of law. Different aspects of the consent process are examined in a number of chapters in this book. This

100

chapter examines consent to treatment in the context of the competent adult patient. The chapter is divided into three main parts. Part one examines the general nature of consent and capacity to consent. Part two is concerned with the liability of the nurse in civil and criminal law if she fails to provide the patient with information regarding her treatment. Part three examines the problem of the nurse who believes that a doctor has given her patient insufficient information with which to make the treatment decision. Some of the difficulties which can face the nurse in attempting to act as advocate for her patient are examined particularly in the context of inter-professional conflicts of disclosure.

6.1 A broad general consent

6.1.1 The consent form

One of the most frequent cries to be heard in a hospital is 'have you got her consent form?'. All nurses are familiar with the consent forms given to the patient to sign before she has an operation. But signing a consent form is not necessary to make that consent legally binding – oral consent may be perfectly valid. However, although written consent may not be strictly necessary the advantage of obtaining written consent is that it draws the patient's attention to the fact that she is consenting to a clinical procedure and it may also provide some evidence of her consent in any future dispute as to whether consent was given.

6.1.2 Express and implied consent

While consent may be given expressly, whether in writing or orally, in some situations even express oral consent is not required. If a patient proffers her arm to the nurse for a bandage to be applied, though she may say nothing her actions imply that she has consented to the procedure. But there are dangers in too readily assuming that a patient has given implied consent. For example, particular difficulties can arise in relation to blood tests. When blood samples are taken a number of tests are usually performed on the samples. It has been argued that by giving general consent to a blood sample being taken a patient is consenting to all those tests being performed which the doctor considers to be necessary [3]. But what if one of the tests is to determine the patient's HIV status? Is this test of a different nature?

It is clear that the implications for a patient if an HIV test is taken are considerable. For example, it may inhibit their ability to obtain insurance and employment. The precise legal position as to whether blood can be tested for HIV without consent remains uncertain. Different legal opinions have been expressed upon this point [4]. Guidance to nurses on testing has been provided by the UKCC. This states that if the nurse takes blood from a patient for the purpose of HIV testing without the patient's consent, or if she co-operates in blood being taken, then she runs the risk of being reported to the UKCC for misconduct [5]. Initially the UKCC unlike the GMC did not recognize any exceptions to this principle. However in guidance issued in 1994 [6] it is stated that in certain 'rare and exceptional' circumstances unconsented testing may be undertaken if this in the interests of the particular patient and it is not possible to obtain consent. This is unlikely to occur in most situations. One possible example might arise if in the future a cure were found and therefore a test would facilitate proper diagnosis and treatment.

6.1.3 *Capacity to consent*

In order for consent to be valid in law a patient must have capacity to make that treatment decision. (See Chapter 8, section 8.2 for the problems of consent and the incompetent patient.) Adult patients are presumed to have capacity to consent or refuse consent to a particular treatment but this presumption can be rebutted (*Re T* (1992)). What is capacity? In a leading case concerning consent and the child patient *Gillick* v. *West Norfolk and Wisbech Area Health Authority* (1985) the House of Lords held that a child patient had capacity if she had sufficient understanding to make that particular decision.

More recently the courts had an opportunity to consider the test of capacity in the context of the adult patient. In *Re C* (1994) the court upheld the right of a 68-year old paranoid schizophrenic who had developed gangrene in his foot to prevent his foot being amputatated in the future without his express written consent. Mr Justice Thorpe suggested a three part test to determine capacity.

- Did the patient comprehend the information given to him?
- Did he believe it?
- Had he weighed up the information balancing needs and risks before reaching his decision?

At the hearing it was claimed that C was not competent because of his delusions that he was a doctor and that whatever treatment was given to him was calculated to destroy his body. But despite these claims Mr Justice Thorpe held that he was satisfied that C was capable of giving or refusing consent because he understood and had retained the relevant treatment information and believed it and had arrived at a clear choice. (See Chapter 9 section 9.3.5 on the question of enforcing advance directives, whether in the form of court orders or patient statements.)

One difficulty with the test laid down in *Re C* is that it makes capacity dependant upon the information which the patient is actually given [7]. If the nurse provides a patient with a great deal of complex information she may be unable to understand it and thus may lack capacity while had she been given a very simple basic explanation about the same treatment procedure she would have possessed capacity.

The Law Commission, a body established by the government to examine areas of law and make recommendations for reform, has suggested a different test of capacity. In their Consultation Paper *Mentally Incapacitated Adults and Decision-Making – Medical Treatment and Research* they propose [8] that a mentally disordered person

> 'should be considered unable to take the medical decision in question if he or she is unable to understand an explanation given in broad terms and simple language of the basic information relevant to taking it, including information about the reasonably foreseeable consequences of taking or failing to take it, or is unable to retain the information for long enough to take an effective decision.'

As the Law Commission note, were such a test introduced into English law most patients would have capacity to consent.

But is this the best approach to take? [9] As Brazier comments [10] an elderly woman with a diseased tooth may have sufficient capacity to understand the suggestion made to her that it should be removed but she may nevertheless allow her fear of dentists and of the pain of treatment to overcome her wish to have the tooth extracted. One way of dealing with a problem patient such as this old lady would be to say that while she may be competent to take some decisions this particular decision is 'irrational' and it should be overridden.

A variation on this approach suggested by Kennedy [11] is that an irrational decision should be respected if it is one derived from long-held beliefs and values on the basis of which a patient has run his life, but not if it was the result of a temporary delusion. However attempting to distinguish between different 'irrational' decisions may be practically very difficult. Furthermore there is a real risk that those refusals declared 'irrational' will be those of the mentally handicapped and the demented patient [12]. It is suggested that the Law Commission are correct when they say [13] that

> 'Many beliefs or value systems have little or no rational basis but we nevertheless respect people's rights to hold them, even to their own detriment ... [T]he issue should be whether the patient is capable of understanding information relevant to the decision.'

6.1.4 *Fluctuating capacity*

Where a patient has a fluctuating mental state it may be acutely difficult to decide whether she is capable of giving consent. In such a situation it is tempting to say she lacks capacity to take treatment decisions. This is because English law allows the incapacitated patient to be given such treatment as those treating her believe to be in her best interests (*F* v. *West Berkshire Health Authority* (1989). In *Re R* (1991) the Court of Appeal held that a child with fluctuating mental capacity was to be regarded as totally incapable of making a decision to consent or refuse consent. However, in the later case of *Re T* (1992) the Court of Appeal held that as far as the capacity of an adult patient is concerned, this is to be judged by reference to the particular decision to be made. This is surely right. If a patient is capable today of understanding what treatment is proposed the fact that yesterday she was not capable of understanding should not affect her right to make a decision.

As noted above, the test of capacity is under consideration by the Law Commission and there is the possibility of future statutory reform. Whatever test for capacity is recognized in law, in practice much will depend upon the discretion of the health care professional. Good practice would suggest that the right of the patient to choose should be respected.

6.2 Consent – criminal and civil law obligations

6.2.1 *Consent and criminal liability*

Bringing a criminal prosecution against a nurse if treatment has been given without a patient's consent may seem an unlikely proposition. Nevertheless, as a recent example graphically illustrates, there may be some situations in which a prosecution may be considered. A 51-year old journalist woke up in hospital after a 'deep scrape' operation to find that during the operation her womb and ovaries had been removed. [14] The surgeon found a swelling in her abdomen, though it was not a life-threatening condition, and had gone on to cut out her ovaries. He said that 'I thought at her age it was the wiser thing to remove them.' The woman took her case to the Director of Public Prosecutions, although it was ultimately decided not to undertake a prosecution.

Where a major operation has been undertaken without consent a prosecution may be brought under section 18 of the Offences Against the Person Act 1861. This section makes it an offence to 'unlawfully and maliciously' cause grievous bodily harm to a person with the intention of causing grievous bodily harm. However it is more likely that a nurse who has given treatment without the patient's consent will be prosecuted for the less serious crime of battery. This makes unlawful any non-consensual touching [15].

As a general rule once a patient has given consent to a medical procedure being undertaken there will be no liability in criminal law. But the fact that consent has been given does not automatically mean that the treatment itself is lawful. English law does not allow a person absolute freedom to do what she wishes with her body (*R* v. *Brown* (1993). Some medical procedures such as female circumcision are expressly prohibited by statute [16] while uncertainty surrounds the legality of others (*Bravery* v. *Bravery* (1954). For example, the legality of animal to human transplantations is still to be resolved [17].

6.2.2 Consent and civil law liability – battery

General principles

While treating without obtaining the patient's consent may lead to a criminal prosecution it is more likely that the patient will bring a claim for damages in the civil courts. First an action may be brought for the tort of battery. An action in battery arises if a patient has been touched without consent. Not every touching will lead to liability, for example an action is unlikely to result from accidently brushing a patient's shoulder as you pass in a corridor. There is no need to prove that the touching caused damaged – the fact that it took place is sufficient for an action to be brought.

In *Chatterson* v. *Gerson* (1981) Mr Justice Bristow held that no liability in battery would arise as long as the patient had been informed and has understood in broad terms the nature of the procedure, and she had given consent. Once a broad general consent has been given, a claim by a patient that she has been given inadequate information should be brought not in battery but in negligence [18].

Treating in an emergency where no consent or refusal can be obtained

There are some situations in which it is lawful for the nurse to go ahead and treat a patient without obtaining consent. If a patient is brought bleeding and unconscious in the early hours of the morning into the accident and emergency department of her local hospital she can be given such treatment as is immediately necessary. If a patient has given initial consent to an operation but then, later, during surgery it is discovered that she is suffering from a life-threatening condition such as a cancerous tumour then this may be removed. But while procedures may be undertaken without consent in an emergency, what is 'necessary' is a matter of degree (*Devi* v. *West Midlands Health Authority* (1981)). The nurse should ask herself if this particular procedure is immediately necessary or could it be postponed until the patient recovers consciousness and can make her own decision.

Respecting refusal of treatment

Just as the patient has the right to consent to medical treatment she has a right to refuse consent. An action in battery may be brought if treatment is given in the face of an explicit refusal of consent. A well-known case often quoted as a warning to those who may be tempted to treat in the face of refusal is the Canadian case of *Malette* v. *Schuman* (1988). The plaintiff was brought into hospital following a road accident. A nurse found a card in her pocket identifying her as a Jehovah's Witness and requesting that she was never to be given a blood transfusion. The nurse gave the card to the doctor treating the patient. Despite the card the doctor performed the transfusion. On recovering her health the patient brought an action in battery against the doctor. She succeeded and was awarded $20,000 damages.

Overruling a refusal of treatment

While a clear refusal should be respected there are situations in which a patient's refusal may be overridden. General guidance for health care professionals was laid down in *Re T* (1992). This case concerned a patient who refused a blood transfusion. This decision had been reached after she had spent some time alone with her mother who was a Jehovah's Witness – T was not herself a Jehovah's Witness. The hospital caring for T sought an order authorizing them, if it became necessary, to administer a blood transfusion to T despite her refusal of consent.

In delivering judgment in this case Lord Donaldson laid down a number of guidelines to assist health care professionals faced with patients who were refusing treatment.

- If a patient had refused consent this could lead those treating him to ask whether he was capable of refusing consent to treatment.

- The implications of treatment refusal vary tremendously and the nurse should consider whether the refusal of treatment means that the patient will only suffer pain and discomfort at one extreme or whether refusal means almost certain death.

- The scope of the refusal should also be considered – whether it applies in all situations, and whether it is based upon assumptions which have not been realized.

- In addition the nurse should consider whether the patient's decision has been reached without undue influence being applied.

In *Re T* itself the court authorized treatment. First, they found that this patient was no longer competent to make the decision to refuse treatment. Second, all the judges in the Court of Appeal stressed the role played by the mother in her daughter's change of heart and that the daughter's will may have been overborne. If a patient refuses treatment when it is clear that without treatment she will die, and if there are doubts as to whether she has capacity to make the decision to refuse treatment, then an application may be made to the court, as in *Re T*. The court is asked to make a declaration, a judicial statement giving guidance as to whether or not it is legal to treat this patient in the absence of consent.

Particular problems in overriding refusal of consent

Refusal of palliative care

A terminally ill patient decides that he no longer wants to continue with a course of therapy and asks for all treatment to be withdrawn so that he can die in peace (see also Chapter 9). The nurse may be placed in a difficult position. As advocate for her patient she may feel that she must respect his wishes. But at the same time she also has to consider the interests of the other patients in the ward. It has been suggested that a patient's right to refuse treatment should not extend to palliative care [19] because of the traumatic effect that their death would have, both for those caring for the patient and for the other patients in the ward, and this issue is presently being considered by the Law Commission. But should the right to refuse be overriden on this basis? Some meet death with terror, some may greet it with joy. A patient refusing palliative care may in fact die peacefully. One instance which was mentioned to the present writer was of a patient who decided to meditate himself to death gradually refusing all medication, food and water.

To require all patients to receive palliative care may also cause distress to the medical staff if a patient who is refusing all care has to be force fed. Very careful consideration needs to be given to these issues before any statutory exception requiring a patient to receive palliative care is introduced.

Pregnant women refusing care

A midwife is faced with a pregnant woman in difficulties in labour but who is refusing even to contemplate a caesarean section. By rejecting treatment she is placing her life and that of the fetus in jeopardy. Should her refusal of treatment be respected?

This issue was brought before the courts in the case of in *Re S* (1992). S was six days overdue giving birth. The medical team wanted to undertake a caesarean section because if a normal birth was attempted it would place the life of both mother and child in grave danger because the fetus was in transverse lie .S, a 'born-again' Christian, refused the operation on the grounds that it was against her religious beliefs. The hospital where she was in labour sought a declaration from the court which was granted by Sir Stephen Brown, the President of the Family Division.

The decision – notable for its haste and brevity – has been criticized [20]. First, in reaching his decision the judge made reference to the rights of the fetus, but English courts have in the past consistently rejected claims that the fetus has such rights (*C* v. *S* (1988) and *De Martell* v. *Merton and Sutton Health Authority* (1992)).

Second, Sir Stephen Brown, in reaching his decision, placed emphasis upon an American case *Re AC* (1990). In a number of cases in the United States courts have ordered a women to be given a caesarean section despite her refusal of treatment [21]. In *Re AC* (1990) the court initially ordered a caesarean section on a woman dying of cancer. This order was overturned on appeal after AC had died. The court said that in 'virtually all cases' a refusal could not be overridden. They did admit there may be exceptional circumstances in which a caesarean may be ordered.

An example given was very similar to the facts of *Re S*. Nevertheless *Re AC* is widely seen as the case which stemmed the tide of judicially-ordered caesareans.

Re S is thus a far from conclusive authority in favour of enforced casearean sections. It can be regarded in many ways as an exceptional case and it is questionable whether the approach taken would be followed in subsequent cases. (See also Chapter 9, section 9.4.3.) There are dangers in using the law to regulate the conduct of women during pregnancy. In the United States [22] court intervention has extended beyond the life and death situation to instances where it was believed that the mother is not taking adequate care of herself during pregnancy.

Were such an approach to be taken in this country it raises what is surely a terrifying prospect of the midwife going beyond advising a woman that certain activities are undesirable during pregnancy to giving warnings of possible legal consequences should she not behave in certain ways. There is even the danger of the midwife being involved in initiating legal proceedings. Serious questions should be addressed as to the scope of professional practice and the nature of fetal rights as against maternal rights before judicial regulation in this area is developed. In this situation should the midwife act as advocate for the mother, or the fetus, or both? The resolution of such difficult issues of public policy should not be left to the courts but should be considered by Parliament, after wideranging public consultation.

Re S was a case which concerned treatment in hospital. What if the pregnant woman refusing care is in her own home? This issue has never come before the courts and the midwife may be in a difficult situation.

She should immediately seek medical advice. It may be possible to persuade the woman to go to hospital for treatment after making clear to her the implications both for her and for the child in her womb. But there is no power in statute or case law to remove a patient to hospital for treatment unless she falls under the Mental Health Act 1983. In forcibly removing the woman to hospital the nurse risks both a criminal prosecution and an action in battery.

Refusal and the dependant family
Can the patient's refusal of treatment be overridden if she has a dependant family? This question has never been brought to an English court but has arisen in the United States where courts have been prepared to uphold the right of a patient to refuse treatment regardless of the impact upon the family *Norwood Hospital* v. *Munoz* (1991). It is suggested that this is the correct approach to take and that, however unfortunate the consequences for the family, if a competent patient has made a clear refusal of treatment this refusal should be respected.

Free (not forced) consent
A patient must make her decision, whether to consent or refuse treatment, freely and without pressure being applied by relatives or by carers. In *Re T* (1992) (discussed earlier in this section) an important factor in the decision to authorize a transfusion was that T's refusal of a blood transfusion came after she had spent time alone with her mother, a confirmed Jehovah's Witness. Ensuring that a patient gives free and full consent may be practically very difficult for a nurse working on a busy ward. Inevitably the amount of time a nurse can spend with a patient discussing the implications of a treatment decision is subject to the constraints of practice, but the patient must not be browbeaten into making the decision.

The fact that a patient is, for example, a prisoner does not mean that she is unable to give free consent. In *Freeman* v. *Home Office* (1984) the court held that whether the prisoner/patient had in fact consented was a question of fact for each individual case. But in this type of situation it is of particular importance that when information is given to the patient it is made clear to her that she has a free choice.

6.2.3 Consent and civil law liability – negligence

For a general discussion on negligence see Chapter 5.

An obligation to disclose?
Obtaining a broad general consent to medical procedures being performed is sufficient to avoid liability in battery. But in addition for a

patient to give a full and effective consent she must have some appreciation of the risks that the medical procedure in question may go wrong. If a patient is not informed of the risk of complications and if one or more of these complications arises then she may bring an action in negligence. The basis of her claim is first that those treating her are under a duty to provide her with information about the risks of the treatment, secondly that this duty has been broken and thirdly that she has suffered harm as had she known of the risk (which in fact materialized) she would not have consented to the treatment.

The leading case is *Sidaway* v *Board of Governors of Bethlem Royal Hospital* (1985). Mrs Sidaway underwent an operation after having suffered for some time from a recurring pain in her neck, right shoulder and arm. The operation was performed by a senior neurosurgeon at the Bethlem Royal Hospital. Even if the operation had been carried out with all due care and skill there was a 1–2% risk of damage to the nerve root and the spinal column. Although the risk of damage to the spinal column was less than to the nerve root, the consequences were more severe. The plaintiff was left severely disabled after the operation. She brought an action in negligence claiming that she had not been given adequate warning of the risks of the operation. During the hearing of the case it was revealed that while the surgeon had told her of the risks of damage to the nerve root he had not told her of the risks of damage to the spinal column. In acting in this way he was conforming to what in 1974 would have been accepted as standard medical practice by a responsible and skilled body of neurosurgeons. The House of Lords rejected the claim that the surgeon had acted negligently. The majority held that the test which a court should use in deciding whether the advice given was negligent was the same as that used in deciding whether medical treatment was negligent, the *Bolam* test. This test provides that a doctor

> 'is not guilty of negligence if he has acted in accordance with a practice accepted as proper by a responsible body of medical men.'

The obligation of disclosure established in *Sidaway* applies to all type of medical procedure. No distinction is drawn between therapeutic and non-therapeutic forms of care as was made clear in the later case of *Gold* v. *Haringey Health Authority (1987)*.

While a nurse will not normally be held negligent as long she conforms with what would be expected from a responsible body of professional opinion the court does have the power to disagree with the level of disclosure deemed acceptable by the professional body. However, a court will only overrule a body of professional opinion in an exceptional situation.

What risks must be disclosed? In *Sidaway* it was suggested that the degree of risk and the seriousness of the consequences if the risk materialized were relevant considerations. Minimal risks – for example a risk of paralysis of less than 1% did not have to be disclosed. However if the treatment posed a serious risk of a major complication such as a 10% risk of a stroke this must be disclosed to the patient.

Withholding information in the patient's interests
While in the majority of cases providing a patient with information about her treatment can be seen as a positive step enhancing her autonomy there may be some situations in which those caring for her believe that giving information may cause her harm. It was suggested in *Sidaway* that some information may be withheld under what is known as the 'therapeutic privilege' where this is in the best interests of the patient. In *Sidaway* Lord Templeman said

> 'some information may confuse other information may alarm a particular patient . . . the doctor must decide in the light of his training and experience and the light of his knowledge of the patient what should be said and how it should be said.'

Any decision to withhold information from the patient must be justified. The nurse must make a very careful assessment of the degree of harm which may be caused to the patient by providing full information.

Informed consent – a better approach?
An alternative approach to the professional practice standard set out in *Sidaway* which has been adopted in a number of other countries such as Australia, Canada and the United States is that of 'informed consent' (*Rogers* v. *Whittaker* (1991) and *Reibl* v. *Hughes* (1980)). For example in the United States case of *Canterbury* v. *Spence* (1972) the court declared that

> 'respect for the patient's right of self-determination on particular therapy demands a standard set by law for the physician rather than one which physicians may or may not impose on themselves.'

Several states in the United States now require a standard of disclosure based upon the information which a 'prudent patient' would expect to receive. In *Sidaway* Lord Scarman who delivered a dissenting judgement supported this approach, saying that the patient should be given such information as a prudent patient would wish to know.

But whether the introduction of a prudent patient test into this country would greatly increase the amount of information which patients would receive may be questioned. Even in the United States it has been suggested that the principle of informed consent has been somewhat blunted as information is withheld from patients by health care professionals claiming 'therapeutic privilege' [23].

Radical reform of the English law of consent to treatment to incorporate an informed consent test along American lines appears unlikely – at least in the near future. However there are indications that the amount of information patients are routinely given about their treatment is increasing. For example, the latest standard consent form issued by the Department of Health provides that the fact that sterilization/vasectomy operations may not render a patient permanently sterile must be drawn to the patient's attention [24].

As Brazier comments [25]:

'From now on it should no longer be possible to rely on "responsible medical opinion" to excuse a failure to explain in all cases the risk of any form of sterilisation failing thus restoring the patient to fertility. The patient's right to and need for that information has been given the unequivocal sanction of the Department of Health.'

It is possible that the professional practice standard of disclosure may become more patient-centered as health care professionals, either voluntarily or under pressure from government, provide patients with more information about their care.

The questioning patient

The nurse may give her patient some explanation of the procedures and potential risks of their treatment but the patient may later approach her and ask for further information. How should she respond?

In *Sidaway* some of the members of the court suggested that if a patient asked direct questions there might be an obligation to provide a full response. Lord Bridge said that

'when questioned specifically by a patient of apparently sound mind about the risks involved in a particular procedure proposed, the doctors duty must, in my opinion, be to answer both truthfully and as fully as the questioner requires.'

But these comments were only suggestions and not binding. The issue of disclosure in response to questions came before the Court of Appeal in the later case of *Blyth* v. *Bloomsbury Area Health Authority* (1987). Mrs Blyth was a qualified nurse. She went into hospital to give birth. After the birth she was given a vaccination against rubella and an injection of the contraceptive Depo-Provera. Mrs Blyth said that she did not want to be given Depo-Provera until she had been told about

proceedings and ultimate dismissal for disobeying the orders of the doctor . In disclosing she takes the risk that her assessment of how much information a patient needs may be wrong. In an extreme case if the patient, unable to cope with the information given, suffers a nervous breakdown an action may be brought against the nurse claiming that her disclosure was negligent. In this situation the court would have to examine whether in disclosing the further information the nurse was acting in accordance with a responsible body of professional nursing opinion.

6.3.4 *Protesting but obeying orders*

Alternatively the nurse may protest to the doctor that the patient has been given insufficient information but, on being told by the doctor to obey orders, she may decide not to take matters further. Would she risk being sued by the patient for her failure to disclose [28]? It is likely that any claim of negligent failure to disclose would be brought against the doctor rather than the nurse. Were an action to be brought against the nurse it might not succeed. Again, the court would examine whether she was acting in accordance with a responsible body of professional nursing opinion.

First, the nurse could claim that she was not negligent as she was simply following doctors orders. In a number of cases concerning negligent treatment (for example *Gold* v. *Essex County Council* (1942)) the courts have been prepared to hold that a nurse was not negligent in her actions because she was obeying orders.

Second, a court may find that the nurse was not negligent because of the fact that she had raised her concerns about the level of information with the doctor. Comparison can be drawn with the negligence case of *Wilsher* v. *Essex Area Health Authority* (1986). In this case Glidewell LJ in the Court of Appeal suggested that an inexperienced doctor might avoid liability in negligence by obtaining advice on the course of action to take from a more experienced colleague. But to apply *Wilsher* would surely be wrong; the nurse is not checking with the doctor because she is inexperienced but because she believes that the doctor acted wrongly.

It remains to be seen however whether either of these arguments would protect a nurse who failed to disclose on doctors' orders. In accepting either argument there is the risk that the court would in effect be affirming that the role of the nurse was subordinate to that of the medical practitioner – medical judgment superior to nursing judgment [29].

In summary the nurse may be torn between her professional ethical obligations and directions given in the course of her employment. As a responsible professional there may be situations in which she will be justified in disclosing information against doctors orders but the courts have not yet had an opportunity to consider any cases in which this has happened. The nurse must make her decision carefully, considering what information has been withheld by the doctor and the reasons why he withheld it.

6.4 Conclusions

Determining whether the patient has given a valid consent or refusal may be one of the most simple tasks that a nurse has to undertake or it may be one of the most complex – leading to conflict with other practitioners treating that patient. The law provides a framework for professional practice to operate but on certain issues her scope of liability remains undecided. Even where legal principles are set out in decided cases the practitioner is left with considerable discretion as to how to act in a particular situation. In the area of consent to treatment, as in other areas, with the development of her role as practitioner and as patient advocate the nurse will be faced with increasingly hard choices.

6.5 Notes and references

Acknowledgment

The author wishes to thank Mr John Murphy and Mrs Maggie Mallik who kindly read through an earlier draft of this chapter. The author takes full responsibility for all opinions expressed and any errors which may remain.

See generally on consent to treatment, Brazier, M. *Medicine, Patients and the Law*, 2nd edn., (Chapters 4 and 5), Harmondsworth: Penguin, 1992; Mason, J.K., McCall Smith, A. *Law and Medical Ethics*, 3rd edn., (Chapter 10), London: Butterworths, 1994; Kennedy, I. 'Consent to Treatment' in Dyer, C. ed. *Doctors, Patients and the Law*. Oxford: Blackwell Science Ltd, 1992; and Dimond, B. *Legal Aspects of Nursing*, (Chapter 7), Hemel Hempstead; Prentice Hall, 1990.

1. In this chapter where the term 'nurse' is used it is used a shorthand for nurse, midwife or health visitor.
2. UKCC, *Exercising Accountability*, Part D, London: UKCC, 1989.
3. Mason, J.K., McCall Smith, A. *Law and Medical Ethics*, 3rd edn., London: Butterworths, 1994: p 232.
4. Sharrad, M., Gatt, I. 'Human Immunodeficiency Virus (HIV) Antibody Testing.' *British Medical Journal* 1987; 295; 911; and Dyer, C. 'Another Judgment on Testing for HIV without Consent.' *British Medical Journal* 1988; 296; p 1791.
5. UKCC, *AIDS and HIV Infection; A UKCC Statement*, London: UKCC, 1988.

6. UKCC, *AIDS and HIV Infection; The Council's Position Statement*, Annex 1 to Registrar's Letter 4/1994, London: UKCC, 1994.

7. Grubb, A. *Medical Law Review* 1994, 2; 1; p 92.

8. The Law Commission, *Mentally Incapacitated Adults and Decision-Making: Medical Treatment and Research* (Consultation Paper No. 129), London: HMSO, 1993; Para 2.12.

9. See generally Gunn, M., 'The meaning of incapacity.' *Medical Law* Review 1994; 1; 8.

10. Brazier, M. 'Competence, Consent and Proxy Consents.' In: Brazier, M., Lobjoit, M., eds. *Protecting the Vulnerable*. London: Routledge, 1991; p 39.

11. Kennedy, I. 'Consent to Treatment.' In: Dyer, C., ed. *Doctors, Patients and the Law*. Oxford, Blackwell Science Ltd, 1992; p 56.

12. Brazier, M. 'Competence, Consent and Proxy Consents.' In: Brazier, M., Lobjoit, M., eds. *Protecting the Vulnerable*. London: Routledge, 1991;

13. The Law Commission, *Mentally Incapacitated Adults and Decision-Making: Medical Treatment and Research* (Consultation Paper No. 129), London: HMSO, 1993.

14. *The Sunday Times* November 1992.

15. Skegg, P.D.C., *Law, Ethics and Medicine*, London: Clarendon Press, 1984; p 32.

16. The Prohibition of Female Circumcision Act 1985, section 1.

17. See Mason, J.K., 'Organ Donation and Transplantation.' In: Dyer, C., ed., *Doctors, Patients and the Law*. Oxford: Blackwell Science Ltd, 1992.

18. See the comments of Bristow J. in Chatterson v. Gerson (1981) and Brazier, M., 'Patient autonomy and consent to treatment: the role of the law.' *Legal Studies* 1987; 7; p 169.

19. Grubb, A., *Medical Law Review 1993*; 1; p 84.

20. Grubb, A., *Medical Law Review* 1993; 1; 2; p 931.

21. See further Kennedy, I., 'A woman and her unborn child; rights and responsibilities.' In: Byrne, P., ed. *Ethics and Law in Health Care and Research*. John Wiley, 1990.

22. Thompson, M., 'After Re S.' *Medical Law Review* 1994; p 127.

23. Myers, D., *The Human Body and the Law*, Edinburgh: Edinburgh University Press, 1990.

24. Department of Health, *A Guide to Consent for Examination and Treatment*, HC(90) (22), London: HMSO, 1990.

25. Brazier, M., 'Revised Consent Forms in the NHS.' *Professional Negligence* 1991; 7; 3; p 148

26 UKCC, *Exercising Accountability*, London: UKCC, 1989.

27. UKCC, *Exercising Accountability*, London: UKCC, 1989; p 10.

28. Montgomery, J., 'Doctors Handmaidens.' In: Wheelar, S., McVeigh, S., eds. *Law, Health and Medical Regulation*. Aldershot: Dartmouth, 1992.

29. See Montgomery, J., 'Doctors Handmaidens.' In: Wheeler, S., McVeigh, S., eds. *Law, Health and Medical Regulation*. Aldershot: Dartmouth, 1992.

B An Ethical Perspective – Patient Autonomy
Ann Bird and *John White*

6.6 Uncoerced consent

The main aim of health care is to enhance the well-being of patients and to minimize harm, that is, to act at all times in the patient's best interests. It is important to patients and to health care professionals that this care should be underpinned by consent and not coercion. Trust, confidence and reciprocity are at the heart of the caring, therapeutic relationship.

The law and the medical profession tend to concentrate on informed consent for surgery rather than other aspects of care – where nursing is more centrally involved – such as drug therapy and invasive procedures like catheterization, which can also be of considerable benefit to patients on the one hand and seriously, even fatally, harmful on the other. Here, even though the law may not require written consent, it is essential that the patient understands and freely agrees to therapy. In order to enhance well-being, it is therefore necessary that consent be uncoerced, informed and rational and that the overall benefit outweighs any harmful effects. It is in the endeavour to balance these requirements in all their ramifications that the moral dilemmas of health care arise – and it is often the nurse–patient relationship which is crucial to their resolution.

Jean McHale's contribution has shown that, except in some emergencies or life-threatening cases, a patient has redress under criminal or civil law if an operation is performed without his or her consent. Consent in itself is not always something which legally exonerates, as where someone consents to a mugger's demand for cash. We are clearly talking about consent freely given. But not all freely given consent legally exonerates, either. If in *Sidaway* v. *Board Governors of Bethlem Royal Hospital (1985)* Mrs Sidaway had freely consented to her operation without being told anything about the risks of damage, the surgeon would have been legally at fault. He needed not only her free consent, but her informed consent, that is her consent given with adequate disclosure of the consequences of undergoing the operation to ensure that she understood these.

In some of the cases which Jean McHale describes, informed consent in this sense comes into the picture, in other cases not. The journalist who objected to the removal of her ovaries was not complaining about the fact that she had not been informed of likely consequences, but about the fact that the changes to her body had occurred without her consent at all.

When we look at the ethical, as distinct from the legal, issues involved in Jean McHale's cases, we need to keep this last distinction in mind. We are dealing with two very different kinds of wrongs.

If someone cuts off someone's waist-length hair without their permission when they are asleep, they have acted improperly, in that they have tampered with the person's body without their consent. The 'rape of the lock', like the removal of the ovaries, can be seen as a kind of assault, and, barring exceptional circumstances like battle, assault has been universally regarded as morally wrong. There is a sound reason backing this consensus: if people were to be left free to assault others at will, life would tend to go badly for all of us, so this kind of behaviour must be prohibited.

Failure to obtain informed consent, raises other issues and brings in further ethical values. What kind of informed consent is required and why do we consider informed consent desirable?

Informed consent is important because it helps people to make informed choices. It presupposes people who are self-determined, that is, who within practical constraints are choosing their own path through life. To be a self-determined, or autonomous, person one needs to have options among which to choose; and one needs to know something of the implications and consequences of choosing this or that. The criterion of determining what the prudent patient ought to know is a good one.

Before looking more closely at what autonomy involves, a caveat about the term 'informed consent' – in one way someone who gives in to a mugger's demand for cash and consents to hand over her purse not only consents but gives her informed consent, in that she *understands* what is at issue, including the likely consequences of not agreeing; yet there is no implication in this case that the mugger has *disclosed* any information to the victim. In this chapter we shall be using the term in the 'disclosure' rather than the more inclusive 'understanding' sense. But it is worth remarking that failure to obtain informed consent where this does *not* involve disclosure may be wrong partly because it does not respect the patient's autonomy, even though this is not necessarily the case. The journalist whose ovaries were removed would have understood without needing to be told what the consequences of their removal would be. If she had given consent, it would therefore have been informed consent in the more inclusive sense. Failure to get her informed consent in this sense was ethically adrift partly for the reason already given, that her body was assaulted, but partly also because it did not respect her status as an autonomous person, determining the major contours of her life: it did not leave her with the choice to take this route or that route, but forced her down a single road.

Informed consent, then, in the sense in which we are using the term which implies that health care staff have disclosed information to the patient, presupposes the ethical value we call personal autonomy. In a society, unlike our own, where people are not seen as self-determiners, but as obedient followers of custom or authority, removing part of someone's body without their informed consent in the more inclusive sense could still be castigated as an assault, but scarcely as an affront to their autonomy. (For more on the different senses of 'informed consent', see Beauchamp & Childress [1].)

6.7 Autonomy

6.7.1 Constraints on autonomy

We must return to the question left hanging above, about what autonomy involves. Autonomous people make their own unhampered decisions about how they are going to live. Autonomy is a matter of degree and some people will be more constrained than others. What sorts of things can constrain? Examples would be:

- having very few options;
- other people, public opinion or the mores of one's society forcing or pressurizing one into a certain path;
- internal (rather than external) constraints like ignorance (hence the importance of *informed* consent), mental illness or physical incapacity.

One factor in the court's decision in *Re T* (1992) to allow the hospital to give the patient a blood transfusion was the pressure which her mother put on her to refuse. In making this decision, it was thus exercised, among other things, by considerations of personal autonomy as opposed to coercion.

In the history of the world, not all human beings have been autonomous. In fact in most societies, as far as we can tell, autonomy as an ethical ideal has been non-existent, people seeing their lives as directed not by themselves, but by gods, tribal custom, slave-masters, or, even in some cases in Europe today (e.g. Spain), by the family. Leaving aside adumbrations in older philosophers, personal autonomy is very much a modern ideal, a pivotal feature of the social and political liberalism which has grown up in certain parts of the world in the last four centuries. Even today there are many groups, even within a liberal society like our own, which do not prize it. The Jehovah's Witnesses in some of the legal cases would be one example. They refuse blood transfusions not because as individuals this is how they have freely decided to live their lives, but because in their view God has forbidden transfusions and they must live as God commands. Given that they prize eternal life above all else – including this present life – it is in their view rational for them to refuse a blood transfusion.

6.7.2 *Autonomy and personal flourishing*

Personal autonomy is related to another, and broader, ethical value – personal well-being (or personal flourishing). A large part of what it is to lead a flourishing life is to be successful in satisfying one's most important desires. Some desires one has are those one would rather be without, like wanting to smoke or drink to excess, or to be spiteful to one's partner. But one can also have second-order desires, that is desires to desire, or not desire, something. The person who wants to give up heavy drinking desires not to desire to drink. His more important desire is to be a person of a certain sort, perhaps one with self-respect, with the energy to throw himself into worthwhile projects. In so far as this person succeeds in satisfying these higher-order desires, his well-being will be increased. Other people may have different central desires – to be of service to others, perhaps as a nurse or a teacher; to lead a comfortable and financially secure existence; to write decent poems.

One can lead a flourishing life without being autonomous. In a tradition-based society where one's major goals are laid down for one – where a man is expected to be a good warrior, father and religious observer and a woman a good wife, labourer and mother, one person may succeed in achieving them, while another, through ill-luck, ill-health or incompetence, may fail. The autonomous life is one version of personal flourishing, especially prominent in societies like our own. For most of us our goals are not laid down by custom or religious authority and we cannot conceive our own well-being except as self-determiners, given, no doubt, that we respect the values of others.

6.7.3 *Autonomy and western society*

An example of the importance we attach to autonomy in everybody's life within the society is found in professional practice towards Jehovah's Witnesses in need of blood transfusions to stay alive. Although they themselves may value obedience to God above autonomy, the law, in allowing them to refuse treatment, is operating on the general assumption that people should not be forced to do what they do not want to do, an assumption that rests in turn on the liberal belief in self-determination.

We value not just autonomy, for that is compatible with its restriction to a few: we see it as an ideal which is applicable to *everyone*, or virtually everyone. In the cases which Jean McHale discussed, the autonomy of the patient was often at issue, as was the autonomy of the nurse. Whatever anyone's situation in life, according to the ideal, one should as far as possible be able to chart one's own way. Patients need to be able to choose whether or not to have treatment. Nurses, having autonomously contracted to do their job, must abide by its requirements;

but when, as in Jean McHale's account, they believe that the amount of information a doctor is prepared to give to a patient is not adequate and would like to be involved in decisions about disclosure, it is the value of autonomy that comes into play. As autonomous persons, nurses do not blindly follow orders or adopt the pronouncements of senior staff: they insist that these conform to ethical values which are of major concern to them, not just as nurses but as human beings – in the situation under discussion, the value concerned is the personal autonomy of the patient and the need for full information about options that this brings with it.

6.8 Autonomy in health care today

In this way, the autonomy of the nurse and the autonomy of the patient are becoming increasingly interdependent, in that moves to encourage the one often also encourage the other. One of the central aims of nursing education today is the development of autonomous practitioners who are better able to assist patients to cope and to take decisions. And with the advent of the 'named nurse' for each patient in the Patient's Charter, the modern nurse practitioner has a key role in helping the patient to give informed consent.

The nurse, whether based in hospital or the community, is usually involved in her patients' everyday world and this enables her to appreciate, from the patients' perspective, how the latter perceive events, what meaning these have for them and where things come in their scale of values. This is important because the major upheaval of illness or disability means that significant adjustments have to be made by patients and their families. These may drastically affect the patients' occupations, personal relationships, indeed whole way of life. Health care professionals need to understand from within how patients' perceptions and value-priorities are affected, and here the nurse's role is crucial.

In order to secure informed consent it is sufficient in law that a patient is told 'in general terms' what treatment is involved. From the moral perspective, however, it is essential that the patient correctly grasps the implications of the various options, their beneficial and probable harmful effects, significant risks and consequences for one's person, lifestyle and projects. It is here that the nurse plays a central role in assisting the patient in making correct interpretations and appraisals.

There are several situations where, for different reasons, the patient's capacity to make informed choices may be at risk and where nurses can help.

Modern western society, as we have seen earlier, is concerned with providing an adequate range of options in different areas. In a publicly funded health service, however, very few options may in fact be available for patients. They have to attend the hospital which has a contractual agreement with their GP; and this could be anywhere in the country and offer only those options which a particular surgeon is willing to provide. It may be very difficult to change to another consultant who is skilled at providing the patient's preferred treatment package. In this case it might be in the best interests of the patient to consent to the treatment that the surgeon and team are most skilled at providing.

Recently some patients urged their surgeons to use micro-surgical techniques so as to shorten their hospital stay. The surgeons, following this sustained pressure, reluctantly carried out the operation which the patients preferred. But since they were not so skilled in this, complications followed, to the patients' detriment. Where the range of options is less than satisfactory in this way and cannot sensibly be enlarged, the nurse can help patients, in talking things through with them, to make the most reasonable choices in prevailing circumstances.

A second example: it is normally taken as read that a patient's questions be truthfully answered, but sometimes problems arise because patients do not ask pertinent questions in the first place. Sometimes this is because they lack the requisite knowledge, but sometimes it is because they are so stunned and frightened at the prospect of a diagnosis of a severe or life-threatening disease that they do not want to ask important questions and may only express trivial worries. From a moral point of view, health care professionals must provide all the appropriate information required by a prudent patient to make an informed choice, even if this is not asked for. In their day-to-day contact with patients, nurses are, once again, in a good position to assist in this, helping to overcome the psychological obstacles on the patient's part to hearing what they need to know.

They may also be in a good position to help where a patient autonomously chooses the option that appears the most harmful from the perspective of the experienced and knowledgeable practitioner, such as refusing life-sustaining treatment when the prognosis is in fact good. After all, beneficence – i.e. the promotion of other people's interests – is as central a value in health care as autonomy: there is a thin dividing line between respecting a person's autonomy on the one hand, and not being open to the charge of negligence, or failure of duty to care, on the other. In cases like this, where accountable nurse practitioners are in serious doubt about what it is best to do, they can seek guidance from the courts.

Dilemmas can arise for the nurse when, for example, the well-being of the family conflicts with the decision of a patient who is rather slow on the uptake or 'pigheaded'. A case in point could be an aggressive patient who constantly abuses his wife. He refuses oral sedation even though he acknowledges that the drug is good for him. The family pressurizes the nurse to put the sedation in the patient's coffee, this being the action they take at home in order to protect his long-suffering and ailing wife. Should the nurse carry out the patient's instructions or act to maximize well-being and minimize suffering on utilitarian considerations?

A final example has to do with the fragmentary nature of the information that patients often have on the basis of which to make choices. They can be told different (not necessarily conflicting) things by various health care professionals on different occasions; and they also bring with them beliefs based on their own past experience, present perceptions and hearsay. Unco-ordinated information of this sort can leave patients bewildered and cloud their understanding. The emotionally disturbed patient may, furthermore, not absorb or quickly forget what is said to them. Again, the nurse should at all times encourage the patient to share his or her perceptions, so that these can be clarified and integrated into a coherent set of beliefs.

In all these ways nurses can be of benefit to patients in coming to informed choices. But nurses do not act on their own. As we have just mentioned, various other health care professionals give patients information. As we have seen, moral difficulties may arise for nurses who consider that crucial information has been withheld by medical staff. In a recent case in the United States, a nurse was disciplined because she told the patient what she thought he ought to know, the surgeons arguing that the information divulged was not within the nurse's remit. The absence of clear boundaries between professional roles and competences make things difficult in such cases.

The conception of the multi-disciplinary health care team should in theory help to overcome this problem. But it may generate problems of its own. One of these arises from the institution of 'advocacy.' When this is conceived in an adversarial way, it can cause disharmony within the multi-disciplinary team. Another difficulty concerns the place of individual moral obligation when this conflicts with the collective decision-making of the team – when for example a 'do not resuscitate' decision is made by the team without the consent of the patient, while the nurse believes that the patient can benefit by resuscitation. Here the UKCC guidelines described in section 6.3.1 are invaluable.

6.9 Autonomy in society

Why is autonomy, if it is, a good thing? It is not necessarily good for everybody: as we have seen, one can lead a flourishing life without it. Some would also say that in our kind of society we can have too much autonomy. Think of all those endless options that oppress us all at times when trying to choose where to go on holiday, how to furnish our flat, even what to select from a menu. But the fact, if it is a fact, that there can be too many options, does not imply that we would be better off without autonomy at all.

In our kind of society, many of the institutions among which we live themselves presuppose that people will be making autonomous choices. In the main, in the UK, marriages are self-determined, not arranged; people choose their jobs and place of residence rather than being directed to them by the state as in some totalitarian countries; our democratic political system presupposes that every citizen has in theory an equal say in determining the broad lines of policy.

Closer to home, the insistence on informed consent to medical treatment also presupposes, as we have seen, that patients are to be seen as autonomous persons. All these institutions – and others besides – can be labelled 'autonomy supporting institutions'. They so pervade our social world that it would be very difficult for anyone to flourish in mainstream society unless they had been brought up to be autonomous. In this way the justification of autonomy goes back to personal flourishing. Not everyone needs to be autonomous in order to flourish, but for us in our kind of society, where the conventional expectation is that people choose their own sexual life-style, partner, job, home, leisure interests, religious (or non-religious) orientation, we would find it difficult to achieve a flourishing life unless we had autonomous propensities.

6.10 An alternative view

The account that we have given of autonomy and why it is valuable is different from that of Gerald Dworkin, who has also written about informed consent to medical treatment and sees this as having its roots in autonomy [2]. For Dworkin autonomy is a characteristic of all human beings, not just those living in a liberal society like our own. Key to autonomy, for him, is the second-order ability we mentioned earlier to reflect on one's desires and to sift them through and act on them or reject them according to their worthiness in one's life as a whole. All human beings possess this ability to form higher-order desires. A consequence of Dworkin's analysis, which he accepts, is that 'someone who wishes to be the kind of person who does whatever the doctor orders is as autonomous as the person who wants to evaluate those orders for himself' [2].

This is at odds with the position we have been taking here, where autonomy is above all to do with self-determination rather than other-determination. In our terms, Dworkin's account is closer to what we have been calling personal well-being, or flourishing. The person whose considered major desire is that her doctor, her mother, God, the state make her important decisions for her may flourish better if that desire is satisfied. But such a person is far from autonomous in our terms. On specific occasions one can, of course, autonomously decide to accept the decision of a wise person or one who is more competent than oneself; but doing *whatever* someone else tells one to is not – in our view – to act autonomously at all.

Not surprisingly, Dworkin's account of why autonomy is valuable is also different from ours. Whereas we have claimed that autonomy is important only for people such as us in our kind of culture to enable us to flourish better, Dworkin has to show why for any human being autonomy is a good thing. His reason seems to be that 'autonomy is a capacity that is (partly) constitutive of what it is to be an agent' [2]: in other words, it is so deeply embedded a feature of human nature (unlike that of other animals), that one could not conceive human existence without it.

6.11 Autonomy in social context

Dworkin's view fails to bring out why informed consent is so important. He may well be right in saying that it is characteristic of all human beings that they are authors of their lives in that they prioritize their desires. This may well be true of a member of a prehistoric tribe as it is true of us. But tribal members work out their priorities within a severely delimited framework, set by the mores of their group. Informed consent is needed from patients not because they are human agents like any other, but because, as self-determining persons, they live in a world of options in every major department of life and in the health care area, as in every other, must have adequate understanding of what taking this or that option would involve.

Because this view of informed consent emphasises *individual* self-determination, some people from different cultural and religious traditions may have a great deal of difficulty in accepting it. For example, in one case it was necessary for an Islamic Sudanese woman to have a therapeutic abortion because of possible harm to her life. Although she understood the options and consequences, she refused to give consent until her husband had given his. It was explained to her that it was unnecessary in UK law for husbands to consent. She, however, insisted that whatever the letter of the law, and despite the urgency of the situation, she would not consent until her husband had done so. Unfortunately, the husband could not be traced and by then the woman's life was considered to be in jeopardy. The surgeons invoked 'necessity' to save the woman's life in an emergency and went ahead with the operation without her consent. Nurses felt that the surgeons should have tried harder to trace the husband, as there would be repercussions for the woman's well-being when she was reunited with him.

6.12 Exceptions to the requirement for informed consent

This case also raises the question of whether there are valid exceptions to the principle that informed consent should be sought. Dworkin argues [2] that there are four types: emergency, incompetence, waiver and therapeutic privilege. From a moral point of view, informed consent need not be sought when

- a patient cannot give consent because emergency treatment is necessary;
- for example the patient is psychotic, senile, an infant or otherwise not in a position to consent;
- the patient has asked the doctor not to consult him or her about the course of treatment; and
- the doctor decides that obtaining informed consent would be harmful to the patient.

Two of these, the first and the last, come into sections 6.2.2 and 6.2.3 and an aspect of the second is considered in Chapter 8. Whether or not we should follow Dworkin in seeing all these as exceptions to seeking informed consent, as distinct from merely free consent, goes back to the issue raised in section 6.7.

As we see it, consent can be omitted in emergency cases because one assumes that patients would rate the saving of their life above the uninvited maiming of their bodies. One can imagine such a rule applying even in non-autonomous societies – although there may be complications, as in the case of the Sudanese woman discussed above, where the patient's preferences are not the only ones which count. But the plea of therapeutic privilege has specifically to do with the withholding of information and is thus more intimately linked with issues of autonomy.

Dworkin is in general wary about this plea but does hold that there are some cases where it is clearly justified – e.g. where, as in *Canterbury* v. *Spence* (1972) it was invoked on the grounds that giving the patient full information would have made him too ill or emotionally distraught to make an informed choice about treatment. Dworkin sees this as a case where autonomy is denied in the interests of the autonomy of the patient and he appears to think it a justified exception for this reason. This seems an odd argument, since it is not as though the treatment was undertaken in order to promote the patient's autonomy and neither did it result in that. If therapeutic privilege is ever justified, this must be when it appeals not to autonomy to override autonomy, but to a quite different value, that is, to avoiding a serious threat to the patient's interests.

It would seem that no ethical value is absolute in the sense that it can never be overridden by another value. Autonomy is no exception. There might be occasions, as in the example just given, where respect for autonomy is outweighed by a concern for the patient's basic interests.

This kind of appeal assumes that there are certain things which are in everybody's interests, such things as survival or avoiding agonizing pain. In general this is so, and there may be cases where doctors could reasonably assume that the patient would, if able to do so, agree that such things were in his or her interests also. But the appeal has to be exercised very cautiously. Even though in general it may be part of people's flourishing to avoid death or agony, it may not be true in all cases. Some people would prefer to die than face the consequences of some forms of treatment. There is a danger that the plea of therapeutic privilege may conceal an unjustified paternalism, that is, that the doctor may in all good faith believe, for example, that avoiding death is in the patient's interests, whereas in fact she might be wrong.

Due recognition of the importance of the patient's autonomy should make one wary not only about invocations of therapeutic privilege in general, but also about the weight that should be put, as in the *Bolam* test, on acting 'in accordance with a practice accepted as proper by a responsible body of medical men', as a defence against negligence in matters of informed consent. The appeal here is to professional authority. But such appeals, while commonplace in more authoritarian cultures, have no place in a liberal society premissed on personal autonomy. It is not enough to accept a practice as proper merely because a body of medical men say it is. One needs to know *why* it is held to be proper; in other words, one needs to get at the values, if they exist here, which could outweigh autonomy. The grounds for professional judgments need to be spelt out: it may in some cases be enough to invoke a threat to life as a reason for by-passing informed consent; but, as Lord Scarman in *Sidaway* implied in his judgment, it is never enough to invoke mere authority.

6.13 The future

As the central place of patient autonomy in medical decisions comes increasingly to be recognized, one may look forward to the widening of options that this will bring in its train. Current debates about euthanasia are very relevant here. Some patients, when fully informed about options A and B may find each of them so unthinkable that, if possible, they would prefer to die: if offered option C, an assisted death, they would choose that. As the law now stands, option C is not available. This restricts the autonomy of the patient as it leaves him or her with only two equally unpalatable choices. In the more liberal age into which medicine is now moving, we may hope for wider options, of this and other sorts.

Nurses and doctors are unlike parents and school teachers in that they are not concerned with the initial development of an individual's autonomy, only with its maintenance or reinstatement. But from a wider social perspective they have their part to play in the civic task of trying to ensure that this liberal value is embodied more effectively in our institutions than it is at present. By reducing the bypassing of informed consent to a minimum and by no longer brooking mere appeals to authority, they are helping to turn hospitals and the health service in general into autonomy-supporting institutions and thereby making this value more entrenched in our way of life as a whole. It is imperative that medical practitioners and the law acknowledge the key role that nurses play in achieving informed consent for the sake of patients' well-being.

6.14 Notes and references

1. Beauchamp, T.L., Childress J.F. *Principles of Biomedical Ethics*, Oxford: Oxford University Press, 1989: pp 76ff
2. Dworkin, G. *The Theory and Practice of Autonomy* (especially Chapter 7 on 'Autonomy and informed consent'), Cambridge; Cambridge University Press, 1989.

Chapter 7
Resources and Professional Accountability

A   The Legal Perspective
Robert Lee

Arguments rage about the availability of resources for health care. In spite of government protestations concerning efficiencies gained by health care reforms in the NHS, it is apparent that delivery of medical services takes place in a climate of resource constraint. The purpose of this section is to examine the legal problems which may arise for the nurse in attempting to provide patient care and maintain professional standards under such economic pressures. Amongst the issues considered are the possible allowances made by the courts if nurses are asked to perform duties which outstrip their competence or qualifications, and the options for the nurse faced with such a request. In order to consider this, it is necessary to explain the standard of care demanded by the law.

7.1   Standards of care

All nurses owe their patients a duty of care [1]. Liability is likely to follow if that duty is breached [2]. A breach will consist of a failure to meet the requisite standard of care. Famously, that standard is determined by the *Bolam* test – 'the standard of the ordinary skilled man exercising and professing to have that special skill' [3]. This standard is objective. This is a well-established principle and was reiterated in the House of Lords in *Whitehouse* v. *Jordan* (1981) [4], on appeal from a judgment of Lord Denning in the Court of Appeal which seemed to propound 'the near infallibility of clinical judgment' [5]. Lord Edmund-Davies stressed that if a surgeon (as it was in that case) fails to meet the *Bolam* standard in any respect – even whilst within the exercise of clinical judgment – then the surgeon must be adjudged negligent. He cited with approval the *Bolam* test as applied in the decision of the Privy Council in *Chin Keow* v. *Government of Malaysia* (1967).

'[W]here you get a situation which involves the use of some special skill or competence, then the test as to whether there has been

130

negligence or not is not the test of the man on the top of the Clapham omnibus, because he has not got this special skill. The test is the standard of the ordinary skilled man, exercising and professing to have that special skill.'

The objectivity of the standard is crucial. The law will take no account of human failings in determining whether or not there has been a breach of the duty of care. Within any walk of life, people differ in their capacity to discharge a job. Some are more innovative or energetic; others more thorough or painstaking. However, in imposing an external and objective standard, nurses are given some protection. Thus, there may be a reason why the nurse failed to meet the required standard – tiredness or inexperience for example. Nonetheless, negligence can and will be found. No-one need suggest that the nurse acted in bad faith. Decisions taken in good faith may lead to liability if the objective standard of skill and care is not met [6]. Equally, it will matter not that any failure is a single lapse in a long and trouble-free career. Liability may follow.

The point is well made in the judgment of Lord Justice Mustill in case of *Wilsher* v. *Essex Area Health Authority* (1986) in which he speaks of the possible liability for injuries to a premature baby:

'If the unit had not been there, the plaintiff would probably have died. The doctors and nurses worked all kinds of hours to look after the baby ... For all we know, they far surpassed on numerous occasions the standard of reasonable care. Yet it is said that for one lapse they ... are to be found to have committed a breach of duty.'

It follows that medical personnel may be expected to perform at a standard which, in the circumstances, they would find difficult or impossible to meet. In the words of Brazier [7]

'a doctor who carries on beyond the point when fatigue and overwork impair his judgment remains liable to an injured patient. The fact that the doctor was required by his employer to work such hours will not affect the patient.'

This raises a host of issues. In *Johnstone* v. *Bloomsbury Health Authority* (1991), the Court of Appeal held that the defendant health authority could require junior doctors, by an express term in their contract, to work an average of up to 48 hours per week overtime. However, in exercising its discretion to require that overtime working under the contract, the health authority could not load work onto the plaintiff to such a level that it was reasonably foreseeable that his health might be damaged. This, however, does not answer a second problem which is whether medical practitioners, who feel that the work structure is such that adequate care cannot be delivered to the patient, may then refuse to work further without incurring the risk that they would be held to be in breach of their contract of employment.

7.2 The problem of inexperience

One problem facing nurses is that much of their training is on-the-job. In the case of *Wilsher*, a junior and inexperienced doctor, wishing to monitor the oxygen in the bloodstream of a premature baby, mistakenly inserted a catheter into a vein rather than an artery. Sir Nicolas Browne-Wilkinson V-C accepted in that case that, under ordinary principles of *Bolam*, it would be generally futile to plead inexperience as a reason for failure adequately to provide specialist or technical medical services, since fault would lie in embarking upon the course of treatment in the first place. However, where, as in the instant case, a first year houseman is required to acquire the necessary skill and experience in order to qualify further, 'such doctors cannot be said to be at fault if, at the start of their time, they lack the very skills which they are seeking to acquire.'

This led Sir Nicolas Browne-Wilkinson V-C to suggest that the standard should be fixed by reference to the post occupied by the person in question. Otherwise, 'the young houseman, or the doctor seeking to obtain specialist skill in a special unit would be held liable for shortcomings in treatment without any personal fault on his part at all'. He went on to argue that liability in English law rests upon personal fault so that liability should only follow if the acts or omissions of medical personnel fell short of their qualifications or experience.

This might give some consolation to nurses for it would mean that placed in situations in which their lack of experience exposed them to the threat of legal action, they could plead such inexperience and argue that they met the duty placed upon them personally. However, this judgment omits a vital part of the *Bolam* test and the majority of the Court of Appeal rejected it as a correct formulation of the law. The Court stated that the standard of care must be set in accordance with the special skill which the person professes to have. The patient is generally in no position to enquire whether (e.g.) a nurse actually possesses such a skill, hence the objectivity of the standard. If nurses hold themselves out to the patient as competent to undertake a particular procedure, a duty of care will arise and will be breached if the procedure is negligently performed.

Sir Nicolas Browne-Wilkinson's suggestion of a requirement of personal fault has appeared in earlier cases on medical malpractice [8]. It is worth noting where it leads. It would introduce a subjective standard, and in so doing might lead to the problem for nurses that a finding of liability would constitute a mark of personal failure. Whatever the perception of a medical negligence claim, fault is judged by an objective standard, and persons found liable may not actually be at fault. In moving the standard towards gross negligence Browne-Wilkinson's formulation would make it harder also for the patient to recover compensation for injury.

This, in part, may explain why the two other judges in the Court of Appeal preferred a more traditional pronouncement of the *Bolam* test. In the view of Lord Justice Mustill the duty ought not to be assessed in accordance with the actor performing the duty, rather with the act performed. The standard should be set according to the post occupied. In the words of the judge:

> 'the standard is not just that of the averagely competent and well-informed junior houseman . . . but of such a person who fills a post in a unit offering a highly specialised service.'

Lord Justice Glidewell substantially agrees with this, saying that:

> 'In my view, the law requires the trainee or learner to be judged by the same standard as his more experienced colleagues. If it did not, inexperience would frequently be urged as a defence to an action for professional negligence.'

The wording of both of these formulations is a little loose, but both are clearly intended to indicate that where a person holds out as possessing the requisite skill to provide a particular service, then the standard will be set in accordance with the reasonable skill of the average competent professional ordinarily providing that service.

7.3 Risk and precautions

Although the standard itself is 'objective and impersonal' (per Lord MacMillan in *Glasgow Corporation* v. *Muir* (1943)), the circumstances in which it is exercised will be highly relevant in determining breach. This is well illustrated by a Canadian authority *Moore* v. *Large* (1932). The case concerned the alleged negligence of a doctor who had failed to X-ray the shoulder of a patient following that patient's fall so that a dislocation of the shoulder was overlooked. The Court could find no negligence:

> 'It has not surely come to this that if the cause of the trouble is not apparent to the eye of the surgeon or physician he must advise an X-ray or take the consequences to his reputation and to his pocket for not having done so. Is the X-ray to be the only arbitrator in such a case

and are years of study and experience to be cast aside as negligible?' [9]

This would probably not be so today, but what has changed is not the availability of X-ray (it was available in 1932) but societal expectations of the use of this device in checking against the risk of a particular disorder. To take an X-ray in such circumstances would now be almost standard practice although interestingly, with the link with cancer, attitudes are changing again. Further, the acknowledgment of the risk and any negligence in disregarding it are judged by the standards of the time of the incident and not when any case comes ultimately to court. As Lord Denning said in *Roe* v. *Ministry of Health* (1954), a case concerning contaminated anaesthetic:

> 'He did not know that there could be undetectable cracks, but it was not negligent for him not to know it at that time. We must not look at the 1947 accident with 1954 spectacles.'

This raises the question of how a breach of the standard of care may be determined.

Generally, it will require some balance between the good which the practitioner seeks to achieve by intervention and the risks run by a particular course of conduct in the light of the availability of precautions or safeguards. This may be illustrated by the case of *Mahon* v. *Osborne* (1939) in which there was seemingly obvious negligence in terminating an operation without removing a swab which was left under part of the liver and which caused a complication which eventually resulted in the death of the patient. Lord Justice Scott was prepared, however, to recognize circumstances 'where the patient has been taking the anaesthetic badly, and is suffering from shock' such that the doctor is anxious to terminate the operation and exercises discretion so that 'as soon as he has completed the removal of all swabs of which he is at that moment aware, he asks the sister for the count, and forthwith starts to close the wound'. In the judge's view, a finding of negligence would not be inevitable in such a situation. Here, the importance attached to preserving the life of a patient might outweigh the risk inherent in hastening the swab count.

It is possible to envisage a wide variety of situations within which risks, ordinarily intolerable in good medical practice, are run in situations of dire emergency. In the words of Lord Justice Mustill in *Wilsher*:

> 'full allowance must be made for the fact that certain aspects of treatment may have to be carried out in ... "battle conditions". An emergency may overburden the available resources, and, if an individual is forced by circumstances to do too many things at once, the

fact that he does one of them incorrectly, should not likely be taken as negligence.'

Note that the absence of resources is not of itself a defence, but the fact of the emergency may change the circumstances in which nursing is conducted to the point that if an ordinarily competent nurse might reasonably have made a particular error under such pressure then the court will not find negligence. This is well illustrated by a case from Manitoba, *Roydon* v. *Krasey* (1971) in which a doctor examined an intoxicated patient in a lorry at 1 AM in the morning with the aid of a torch. There was no negligence in his failure to diagnose injuries to the chest, ribs and lungs. One way of explaining this is to say that, under an objective standard, the difficulties in discharging the duty of care would have faced any practitioner working under such circumstances.

7.4 Staff shortages

This then raises the question of what will happen if, in the course of medical practice, a nurse is required to work under substandard conditions, or with an obvious shortfall in resources. Can such circumstances be taken into account in assessing breach of duty? In the following section, which considers shortages of nursing staff, the problem of inexperience will not be revisited, rather attention is directed here to problems created by overall shortages in the nursing resources required to discharge the needs of the patients.

There are a series of cases concerning the provision of nursing staff, many of which involved relatively straightforward issues of patient supervision. *Dryden* v. *Surrey County Council* (1936) is a case involving two elements of medical negligence – one involved the failure to remove a swab, leading to a finding of negligence against the surgeon. However, an action was also brought against the Council on the basis that the nurses, whom they employed, had failed adequately to supervise the plaintiff, so that the error went unnoticed. This element of the claim seems to have been rejected by the court on the basis that, as a matter of evidence, the plaintiff failed to exhibit symptoms which might have indicated a complication of this type. Nonetheless, the court did consider that element of the claim which argued that the responsibility of the Council lay in their failure to provide competent nursing staff as the ward was clearly understaffed. In fact, there were 54 beds in the ward and a nursing staff of one sister, one staff nurse and five probationers. This, as the judge admitted in a masterful piece of understatement, was not as good as 'the attention which a person will receive ... if ... he is fortunate enough to pay for the undivided attention of one nurse or ... two nurses'. However, in the view of the judge, neither the presence of such a large number of probationers, nor the fact that the

Matron had been seeking to gain an increase in staff established 'negligence by understaffing'.

This, at first glance, may seem rather surprising. In fact, however, it may be saying little more than, whatever the level of staff, there will be no finding of negligence unless some injury can be attributed to the lack of nursing care. Where this is so, the court will be required to consider the level of nursing provision. This must be done for the particular ward in question, for once again the courts are dealing with risk of injury, and the nursing provision required in an intensive care facility may not be that of the ante-natal unit (*Knight* v. *Home Office* (1990)).

This point may be demonstrated by cases in which known suicide risks have injured or killed themselves following admission to hospital. In *Thorne* v. *Northern Group Hospital Management Committee* (1964) the patient's husband had informed the nursing staff of his wife's threats of suicide, and the patient, who had been undergoing treatment on a medical ward of a general hospital, was due to be transferred from the ward to an outside neurosis unit for further assessment. She was left unsupervised when both the nurse and the sister left the ward together. The patient left the ward, returned home and committed suicide. The husband failed in his action against the hospital management committee. In the view of Edmund Davies Mr Justice:

'The duty owed by hospital authorities and staff to a patient is that of reasonable care and skill in the given circumstances. Whether a breach of that duty has been established depends on the proven facts including what was known or should have been known about a particular patient and the fact that the defendants impliedly undertook to exhibit professional skill and administrative care of reasonable competence and adequacy towards their patient. They must take reasonable care to avoid acts or omissions which they can reasonably foresee would be likely to harm the patient entrusted to their charge; but they need not guard against merely possible (as distinct from reasonably probable) harm. On the other hand the degree of care which will be regarded as reasonable is proportionate both to the degree of risk involved and the magnitude of the mischief which may be occasioned to the particular patient in the absence of due care.'

This case may be contrasted with that of *Selfe* v. *Ilford and District Hospital Management Committee* (1970) in which the plaintiff, whose attempt at suicide by a drug overdose had failed, was admitted to a ward of 27 patients. The ground floor ward contained four known suicide risks – grouped at one end of the room. Selfe, a quiet and withdrawn man of 17 was left unattended on the ward when two of the three nurses on duty left the ward without informing the third. While that nurse was attending a patient elsewhere in the ward, Selfe climbed out of a window, and made his way up to a roof from which he jumped. His attempt at suicide again failed, but he sued for his resultant injuries on the basis of negligent nursing supervision. Evidence indicated that, even with all of the nurses on the ward, an additional nurse was probably required. Mr Justice Hinchcliff found for the plaintiff, stressing that the high degree of risk on the ward required a commensurate increase in the care provided.

7.5 Lack of resources

Once a finding of fact is made that provision is in some way inadequate, a related issue arises of whether it can ever be a defence to plead lack of resources. The answer is simply no. If nursing staff meet approved nursing practice to a *Bolam* standard, then this may refute a claim of negligence, but if they fall short of that standard, then, once again, it does not matter why, and lack of resources is no better an argument than that of tiredness or inexperience.

However, in spite of the objective nature of the standard, and the lack of any necessary element of personal fault in a finding of negligence, there is without question a move away from finding medical staff liable in situations in which lack of adequate resources makes it impossible to meet a required standard. This is clear from the judgment of Sir Nicolas Browne-Wilkinson in *Wilsher* in which he poses the following question:

'Should the authority be liable if it demonstrates that, due to the financial stringency under which it operates, it cannot afford to fill the posts with those possessing the necessary experience?'

He goes on to say:

'in my judgment, the law should not be distorted by making findings of personal fault against individual doctors who are, in truth, not at fault in order to avoid such questions.'

One can quibble with this. It is not the law which is being distorted; rather it is the law which is distorting the concept of blame. Nonetheless, this move away from the concept of individual liability on the part of a medical professional, in favour of asking questions about the organization as a whole, is significant, and it is important to understand what it represents.

7.6 From vicarious to direct liability

For many years, the view was taken that hospital authorities were not liable for actions of staff in discharging professional duties. This applied to nurses in the course of medical procedures under the guidance of the doctor whose control was thought to be 'supreme'. However, the hospital authority remained legally responsible to patients for 'purely ministerial or administrative duties' and these included 'attendance of nurses in the ward' (per Lord Justice Kennedy in *Hillyer* v. *St. Bartholomew's Hospital* (1909)). This artificial division, and the concept of control which underpinned it, was difficult to maintain, and in *Gold v Essex County Council* (1942), Lord Greene expressed the view that:

> 'Nursing ... is just what the patient is entitled to expect from the institution, and the relationship of the nurses to the institution supports the inference that they are engaged to nurse the patients ... the idea that ... the only obligation which the hospital undertakes to perform by its nursing staff is not the essential work of nursing but only so-called administrative work appears to me ... not merely unworkable in practice but contrary to the plain sense of the position'.

This case effectively established that a hospital authority would be vicariously liable for the negligence of an employee, such as a nurse. A mistake made by a nurse following the direct orders of a surgeon would probably not give rise to liability, but the surgeon no longer ruled 'supreme' even in the theatre. Following this case, a mistake by the nurse alone might mean that there would be no liability on the surgeon, but that vicarious liability might attach to the hospital authority.

It was established in cases such as *Cassidy* v. *Minister of Health* (1951) and *Roe* v. *Ministry of Health* (1954) that the test for vicarious liability was no longer one of control, but of whether the member of the medical staff was a permanent and integral part of the hospital staff. So fixed and well settled was this body of law, that from 1954 to 1990, under a governmental circular, health authorities defended claims in negligence on behalf of all staff. At date of judgment or settlement, damages would be apportioned, in accordance with the principles of vicarious liability, between the medical defence organization and the health authority. Disputes as to the requisite shares of liability were rare.

In *Cassidy*, however, it had been suggested that certain liabilities might be direct, such that the duty of care could not be delegated 'no matter whether the delegation be to a servant under a contract of service or to an independent contractor under a contract for services'. For some years, this *dictum* of Lord Denning lay as an island of uncertainty in the stormy seas of medical malpractice litigation. In recent times, however, the concept of direct liability has received much greater attention. As Montgomery [10] points out:

> 'In a modern system of healthcare ... the responsibilities of doctors overlap with those of nurses, midwives, managers and others. Direct

liability on the part of the health and hospital authorities may represent an important tool to unravel the complexities of modern health provision.'

Direct liability may have advantages in overcoming problems of where to place responsibility amongst health care teams. Equally, it may assist the law in keeping track of standards, as pressure on resources sees the devolution of tasks to nurses which were previously performed by doctors.

All of this is a way of saying that direct liability may arise out of the failure of structures of health care delivery which have been put in place in order to discharge duties towards the patient. Thus, in *Bull* v. *Devon Area Health Authority* (1989) [11] there was a gap of over an hour between the delivery of a first and a second twin. A significant passage of time prior to the case arriving before the court made it difficult for the defendant health authority to find evidence to dispute the claim of negligence, but Lord Justice Slade nonetheless stated that:

'It is possible to imagine hypothetical contingencies which would have accounted for a failure without any avoidable fault in the hospital's system, or any negligence in its working, to secure Mrs Bull's attendance by any obstetrician qualified to deliver the second twin between 7.35PM and 8.25PM. In my judgment, however, all the most likely explanations of this failure point strongly either to inefficiency in the system for summoning the assistance of the registrar or consultant, in operation of the hospital, or to negligence by some individuals in the working of that system.'

This point is supported also by Lord Justice Mustill, who speaks of a 'finding by the learned judge, amply supported by the evidence, that the system should have been such that the second twin would be delivered as soon as practicable after the first'. In considering the submission that the hospital 'could not be expected to do more than their best, allocating their limited resources as favourably as possible', Lord Justice Mustill makes the following response:

'I have some reservations about this contention, which are not allayed by the submission that hospital medicine is a public service. So it is, but there are other public services in respect of which it is not necessarily an answer to allegations of unsafety that there were insufficient resources to enable the administrators to do everything they would like to do. I do not for a moment suggest that public medicine is precisely analogous to other public services, but there is perhaps a danger in assuming that it is completely *sui generis*, and that it is necessarily a complete answer to say that even if the system in a hospital was unsatisfactory, it was no more unsatisfactory than those in force elsewhere.'

Cases like *Bull* and *Wilsher* demonstrate that there are an increasing number of instances in which there seems to be an organizational failure in the delivery of health care. If a health authority is at fault in the performance of its functions, this may be described as negligence, notwithstanding the difficulty in locating particular employees who might be said to be negligent. Arguably, this is the basis of the decision in the case of *Lindsey County Council* v. *Marshall* (1936), and also other earlier cases such as *Collins* v. *Hertfordshire County Council* (1947), which found negligence 'in the management and control of the hospital'. A number of Commonwealth authorities [12] have also found negligence in the organization of the hospital itself.

Finally, there are two relatively recent cases involving the administration of drugs and blood products. In the Court of Appeal decision in *Blyth* v. *Bloomsbury Health Authority* (1987) [13], the defendant health authority appealed against a judgment of Mr Justice Leonard, in which he found that the health authority was negligent in failing to follow a system put in place to monitor the use of the drug Depo-Provera. The appeal succeeded, the Court of Appeal finding that the judge had reached the decision, not supported by the evidence, that there had been divergence from a system put in place within the hospital. Nonetheless, the Court of Appeal seemed to have accepted that the tests used by Mr Justice Leonard in looking at whether 'on a normal day an effective system existed by which patients could get advice on contraception from those who were equipped with the necessary information to enable them to give it fully', and whether 'exceptionally something went wrong' were acceptable tests within themselves. Implicit in the Court of Appeal's judgment is the necessity for a health authority to ensure that patients within the hospital are sufficiently well counselled in relation to drugs administered.

In *Re HIV Haemophiliac Litigation* (1990), an application by the plaintiff to the court for an order requiring the Department of Health and Social Security (DHSS) to produce departmental documents relating to its policies for the importation of blood products was resisted by the DHSS, on the basis that the plaintiffs did not have a good cause of action either by breach of statutory duty or in negligence. The Court of Appeal gave judgment on the preliminary issue of whether or not the DHSS might be in breach of statutory duty under section 3 of the National Health Service Act 1977, or otherwise negligent in the design of a system to secure the physical health of the people, and the prevention, diagnosis and treatment of illness within England and Wales. This was said to result from its failure to ensure a self-sufficiency in blood, as a result of which haemophiliacs were treated with Factor VIII blood products contaminated with the HIV virus, imported from the United States. The Court of Appeal found an arguable case. In their words:

> 'It is obvious that it would be rare for a case on negligence to be proved having regard to the nature of the duties under the 1977 Act, and the fact that, in the law of negligence, it is difficult to prove a negligent breach of duty when the party charged with negligence is required to exercise discretion and to form judgments upon the allocation of public resources. That, however, is not sufficient . . . to make it clear for the purposes of these proceedings that there can in law be no claim in negligence.'

It seems, therefore, that hospitals may increasingly have to face direct liability for their failure to organize adequate systems of health care delivery. Thus, in an era of resource constraint, if the delivery of health care is inadequate, it may become easier rather than more difficult for the patient to find a remedy. This is not least because the courts have traditionally been very protective of doctors (in particular) and that when negligence alleged is that of the organization, rather than the medical professional, certain obstacles to medical negligence litigation may be removed.

7.7 Case study

The principles considered above can be illustrated by the use of a case study.

N is a sister on night duty and is in charge of a small rural hospital which some time ago closed its accident and emergency facility. Shortly before midnight on a snowy winter's evening, two people arrive by car at the hospital. R says that he has found, on the roadside very near to the hospital, an injured person, V, who accompanies him. V has been the victim of a hit-and-run incident. V is fully conscious, but appears to have been hit in his upper body and may have broken a number of bones. He is also bleeding badly from the head. The nearest accident and emergency facility is ten miles away. There is no doctor currently on duty at the rural hospital which has a sign at the gate advising that there is no accident and emergency unit within the hospital, and that persons wishing for emergency treatment should report to their nearest accident and emergency hospital.

One interesting issue here is whether N must offer treatment to the patient. In *Barnett* v. *Chelsea and Kensington Hospital Management Committee* (1968) three nightwatchmen had vomited continually since drinking tea in the early hours of the morning of New Year's Day. On finishing their shift they presented themselves to an accident and emergency department of a London hospital. They reported to a nurse who telephoned the casualty officer. Without examining the men, he told the nurse to send them home with instructions to call their own doctors in the morning. Five hours later, one of the men died from arsenic poisoning. Although the subsequent claim failed on the lack of proof of causation, it was said that where a person with obvious symptoms of illness presents himself to an accident and emergency department, a duty of care arises so that skill and care should be employed in the diagnosis of any injury.

This is so even though there will be no prior relationship with the patient. However, the general view taken by English law is that 'if a person undertakes to perform a voluntary act he is liable if he performs improperly, but not if he neglects to perform it'. It is for this reason that certain jurisdictions have enacted 'good samaritan' statutes which either place a positive duty on doctors to stop at the scene of an accident, or offer immunity to medical staff who choose to render assistance.

Although there is a statutory duty to provide sufficient accident and emergency services to meet reasonable requirements within a locality, in practice this duty will prove very difficult to enforce before the courts. There is now a significant body of case law which demonstrates that the courts will rarely intervene to review a decision on resource allocation or enforce a claim to be admitted to treatment. Nonetheless, if a non-accident and emergency hospital chooses to admit a patient to treatment, then a duty of care will arise. It follows that, in purely legal terms, N would be free to refuse treatment to V and urge R and V to present themselves to the nearest accident and emergency department. Nonetheless, once N opts to render care and assistance to V, then a duty of care arises and the question then relates to the applicable standard of care. It is clear that liability may result from negligent treatment or advice rendered by N or any failure of communication in providing V with emergency treatment.

However, given that the unit is not an accident and emergency unit, then in accordance with the case of *Roydon* v. *Krasey* (1971) (section 7.3) the circumstances in which treatment is rendered will be taken into account in determining the requisite standard of care. In *Knight* v. *Home Office* (1990), it was said that a prison hospital owes a duty of care to a mentally ill patient which is of a lower standard than that of a specialist psychiatric hospital. In that case, it was said that:

'In making the decision as to the standard to be demanded the court must bear in mind as one factor that resources available for public services are limited and that the allocation of resources is a matter for Parliament ... the facilities available to deal with an emergency in a general practitioner's surgery cannot be expected to be as ample as those available in the casualty department of a general hospital.'

What will prove of importance is that N adequately communicates, to anyone else rendering treatment to V, the steps which she has taken and that she arranges for the necessary specialist care as expeditiously as possible.

7.8 Scarce resources and professional responsibility

Questions relating to the relevant standard of care are also significant for nurses in another context. As is stated above the law demands no more than a reasonable standard of care rather than standards of treatment which are at the cutting edge of medical science. But what should nurses do if they become convinced that patients are facing unacceptable levels of risk because the regime of treatment regularly falls short of reasonable standards? Two problems may arise for the nurse who decides to seek publicity to draw to the attention of the public the inadequacy of the care offered. The first is that the identification of a particular patient may breach principles of medical confidentiality. In addition, any public disclosure might amount to a breach of the contract of employment.

Neither the UKCC's *Code of Professional Conduct for Nurses, Midwives and Health Visitors* nor their Advisory Guidelines on Confidentiality suggest an absolute duty of professional confidence. Although clause 10 of the Code instructs the nurse to 'respect confidential information obtained in the course of professional practice and refrain from disclosure without the consent of the patient ...' the Code does allow for exceptional cases of disclosure upon a court order or where this is necessary in the public interest.

This is in accordance with the general law. In *Attorney General v. Guardian Newspaper (No. 2)* (1990) Lord Goff stated that 'although the basis of the law's protection of confidence is that there is a public interest that confidence should be preserved and protected by law, nevertheless, that public interest may be outweighed by some of the countervailing public interest which favours disclosure.' However, in *X Health Authority v. Y* (1988) any public interest in the disclosure of the fact that two practising doctors were being treated as AIDS patients was outweighed by the general public interest in retaining the confidentiality of AIDS-related information on a patient's file. The High Court in this case intervened to restrain the publication of the disclosure when leaked by employees.

However, in the case of *W v. Egdell and others* (1990) a consultant psychiatrist was employed by a patient's solicitor to prepare a report upon the patient for use in the consideration of the patient's release or transfer from a secure hospital. When no use was made of that report (which highlighted the long-standing nature, not previously drawn to the authorities' attention, of W's interest in home-made bombs) the psychiatrist himself disclosed the report to the medical director of the secure unit. In turn the hospital forwarded the report to the Secretary of State. The Court of Appeal stated that whilst mental patients should be free to seek advice and assistance from independent doctors, nonetheless given the wider public interest in public safety, this form of disclosure by the psychiatrist was thought not to be in breach of any duty of confidentiality.

Thus, although it might be possible to argue that disclosure of patient-related information serves wider public interest in highlighting the decline in the standard of care, this is by no means obvious. Where possible, particular patients should not be identified, or, if this is inevitable, then the nurse should seek the permission of that patient to refer to the particular case.

Nurses should be aware that, if they voice public opinions on the regime of care, disciplinary action may be taken by the employer. This is made much easier by the introduction into contracts of employment of express requirements prohibiting disclosure to the media of matters relating to the working responsibilities of employer and employee. Indeed, it could be argued that, even in the absence of an express clause, implied duties of fidelity might dictate that any public disclosure would amount to a breach of the employment contract. There are now well-documented incidents in which health service employees have faced disciplinary proceedings or dismissal, apparently as a result of complaints concerning shortfalls in the standard of care. Where this leads to the dismissal of an employee, that employee may consider redress by an industrial tribunal. This is unlikely to lead to reinstatement, even where the tribunal finds in favour of the dismissed nurse.

One would hope that disclosure within the health care system would be looked upon as a rather different matter than public disclosure. Certainly, it may be hard to justify the actions of a nurse who goes immediately to the press, without seeking any internal redress of alleged deficiencies. The sad fact is that there seems to be evidence that not every complaint made by a nurse is sympathetically received. Clearly by placing themselves in the role of complainant, certain nurses will make themselves unpopular, and even jeopardize their job opportunities.

Nonetheless, increasingly, there are professional demands made upon nurses. The UKCC Code of Conduct suggests that the nurse *must* report circumstances which could jeopardize standards of practice and also report circumstances in which an appropriate standard of care cannot be provided. Such reporting should be to 'an appropriate person or authority'. Again, the UKCC Code suggests that nurses should 'decline any duties or responsibilities unless able to perform them in a safe and skilled manner'. Increasingly it seems that nurses cannot merely stand by and ignore declining standards of patient care. It is the nurse who is seen as occupying the role as patient advocate, and arguably nurses find themselves under a more direct professional duty to take action in relation to resource shortfalls than do the doctors.

Case Study

W is a night duty charge nurse on a ward for acutely ill patients. She believes that the standard of care for those patients has dropped dramatically due to two events: (1) the withdrawal of one night nurse, on a permanent basis, from ward duty, and (2) the replacement over time of a number of more experienced nurses by junior staff. Matters came to a head when a patient dies in distressing circumstances, in a situation in which W believes was largely a consequence of lack of adequate supervision on the ward.

Under UKCC's Code of Conduct, W here should 'report to an appropriate person or authority, having regard to the physical psychological and social effects on patients and clients, any circumstances in the environment of care which would jeopardize standards of practice'. Similarly it is said that she should 'report to an appropriate person or authority any circumstances in which safe and appropriate care for patients and clients cannot be provided'. W clearly finds herself in this situation, and if the hospital in which she works operates a complaints procedure, then she would be advised to follow that procedure and voice her concerns accordingly. If no response is forthcoming, or if such complaints are swept aside, then W may wish to raise the matter with persons further up the management ladder even through to the chair of the health authority or Trust where that appears to be appropriate. Alternatively, at some point W may wish to have recourse to the 'whistle-blow scheme' run by the Royal College of Nursing (RCN). This is aimed at allowing nurses to write directly and in confidence to the General Secretary of the RCN who can, with the complainant's permission, investigate the matter further.

On a strict interpretation of confidentiality rules it could be argued that the passage of information even between those in the health care system should take place only to serve the treatment of the patient. However, if this principle was to be followed rigorously, investigations into medical accident might be inhibited. The General Medical Council allows that doctors must judge whether it is appropriate to pass on patient information to others within the health care system so that they can perform in their duties. Here the permission of the patient cannot be obtained, and public disclosure might cause distress to relatives. Arguably, however, disclosure within the health care system ought to be permissible. However, further problems may arise, where, instead of effecting any remedy, the disclosure by W leads to further problems at work. If W finds herself the subject of formal disciplinary proceedings, or indeed victimized in some way by line managers as a result of the complaint, how should W react? Unfortunately there is little available remedy here. Arguably this could be a matter for the Health Services Ombudsman. Other than this, the only course available to W may be to resign from the post and seek to claim constructive dismissal. Dismissal proceedings have more than once arisen out of whistle-blowing. Such cases have succeeded, or have been settled. However, they provide little recompense for the loss of a job, and being dismissed in these circumstances may not necessarily make it easy for W to find re-employment.

This course of action may also invite press comment, whether or not W actually instigates this. At this point, W will have to take care to avoid breaching professional confidentiality rules in any statements to the press. However, insofar as W and those giving evidence on behalf of W need to give evidence as to the particular events which led to the complaint, the disclosure will generally be permissible under professional conduct rules. Under the UKCC Code disclosure is allowed 'where required by the order of a court'. This does not exactly cover the situation of a tribunal which will not generally proceed by witness summons or the sub-poena of witnesses. Nonetheless, it is difficult to see that a health authority or Trust would have much success in seeking to restrain by court action the disclosure of information, where that information is being legitimately used to pursue a remedy in an industrial tribunal.

7.9 Conclusion

The changes in the delivery of health care in the NHS are based on a market philosophy. This of necessity has had a dramatic and radical impact not only on the methods of service delivery but also on the demands and expectations placed on various health care professionals and the allocation of resources. The devolvement of responsibility on all levels, financial, administrative and professional, down the line from the hospital administrator to the individual nurse implies that issues surrounding professional accountability and autonomy require closer examination.

This change in the underlying philosophy of the delivery of health care in some ways is running in tandem with the growth of legal problems which may arise for the nurse. Problems arise in attempting to provide patient care and maintain the professional standards expected of the 'ordinarily skilled' practitioner. The changes have had, and continue to have, resources implications. The reduction of resources may increase the instances in which nurses are placed in situations which require them to perform duties which it could be argued are beyond their level of competence or qualification. The development of professional skill and qualification is directly dependent on the training received 'on-the-job'.

If resources are stretched the qualified nursing staff will be fully utilized in the delivery of patient care, with time for training limited. Unrealistic demands may be placed on the student or newly qualified nurse, yet, in the eyes of the law, the standards required will remain objective. The spectre of liability demands that attention be given to demonstrable training for, and the maintenance of standards of, the professional nurse. It will be up to individual nurses to show that their qualifications and training are sufficient to the role and task in each and every situation.

Of necessity, the changes in the NHS will not only have personal and professional implications for the nurse but also implications of a systemic nature. The role of the nurse in relation to the patient as well as to the nurse managers will be tested. The nurse has been seen to be the advocate on behalf of the patient and also accountable to a manager. However, the nurse could possibly be placed in a situation where there is a conflict of interest. Meanwhile the UKCC Code deals with the obligatory reporting by nurses when witnessing poor standards of patient care. Yet at the heart of the matter is the relationship between cost, quality and quantity of treatment which it is not open to the individual nurse to resolve.

7.10 Notes and references

1. See *Barnett* v. *Chelsea and Kensington HMC* [1968] 1 All ER 1068; *Gold* v. *Essex CC* [1942] 2 All ER 237; *Urbanski* v. *Patel* [1978] 84 DLR (3d) 650; Lee, R., 'Hospital Admissions – Duty of Care' *New Law Journal* 1979, p 567.
2. Liability will not inevitably follow for a number of reasons. There may be no resulting damage, or the medical error may not be the causative factor or later injury, or the damage may be too remote.
3. Note the incorporation of this principle into statute: Congenital Disabilities (Civil Liability) Act 1976, section 1(5).
4. see also Deutsch, R.L. 'Medical Negligence Reviewed.' [*American Law Journal*] 1983; 87; p 674.
5. Brazier, M., 'Patient Autonomy and Consent to Treatment: The Role of the law' *Legal Studies* 1987; at p 170, and for a wider review of Lord Denning's approach to standards of care see McLean, S., 'Negligence – A Dagger at the Doctor's Back?' in Robson, P. Watchman, P. *Justice, Lord Denning and the Constitution* Aldershot: Gower, 1981.
6. See *Whitehouse* v *Jordan* [1981] 1 All ER 267 and in the USA, *Demmer* v. *Patt* 788 F2d 1387 (8 Cir 1986).
7. Brazier, M., *Medicine, Patients and the Law*, 2nd edn., Harmondsworth: Penguin, 1992.

8. Most famously by Lord Denning in *Whitehouse* v. *Jordan* [1980] 1 All ER 650.
9. *Ibid* at 183 (quoted by Picard E, *Legal Liability of Doctors and Hospitals in Canada* Carswell 1984).
10. Montgomery, J. 'Suing hospitals direct: what tort?' *New Law Journal* 1987; 137 p 703 in reply to Bettle, J. 'Suing Hospitals Direct: whose tort is it anyhow?' *New Law Journal* 1987; 137 p 573.
11. 2 February 1989 [1993] 4 Med LR 117.
12. see *Commonwealth* v. *Introvigne* (1982) ALJR 749, *Kandis* v. *State Transport Authority* [1984] 154 CLR 672 (both Australian HC) and *Albrighton* v. *Royal Price Albert Hospital* [1980] 2 NSWLR 542 CC.A) o.f. *Yepremian* v. *Scarborough General Hospital* [1980] 110 DLR (3d) 513 which seems to accept this possibility; also Dugdale A. & Stanton K, (1989) *Professional Negligence*, 2nd edn, Butterworths, London, para 22.22, who, speaking of duties to provide treatment under the National Health Services Act 1977, state that 'it is undoubtedly the case that the effect of basing this duty on statute is to ensure that it is non-delegable in its nature.'
39. *The Times* 11 February 1987 (Court of Appeal) quotes which follow are taken from the report at [1993] 4 Med LR 151, 156.

B   An Ethical Perspective – How to Do the Right Thing
David Seedhouse

7.11   Introduction

Health care resources are scarce. This is an unfortunate fact of life. In those cases where there is not enough to go around difficult choices must be made. Sometimes nurses must make these choices. This may mean that they cannot help everyone they would like to support. It may mean that they will not be able to offer as much to each patient as they would ideally wish to do, but this is not a perfect world. In order not to waste resources, and in order to be as fair as possible across the health service, all nurses must be aware that rationing is sometimes necessary. Nurses must recognize these facts; nurses must do the right thing.

This, at least, is the official position: it is held (and fostered) by governments preoccupied by the need to keep health care costs in check [1], by several health economists [2], some of whom devote considerable energy to the production of technical 'rationing formulae'; and it is increasingly (though often grudgingly) accepted by many nurses. Slowly but surely the 'official line' has also come to be believed by many of the general public, who listen to the various experts and – not unreasonably – conclude that if those in the know see the need to ration, then there must indeed be such a need.

But is the official position true? Certainly not everyone accepts it. For instance, it has been argued that the basic duty of any government must be to defend its people against threats to life and safety, and that since in normal circumstances health care does this much better than any other sort of public provision (and is infinitely more useful than an idle army), governments must – as a matter of obligation to their subjects – switch military funding to health services [3]. It is also claimed that in the United States, where spending on health care currently consumes around 14% of the gross domestic product, there are already more than enough health services to go round – the problem is that not everyone who needs them can get access (millions of Americans do not have health insurance, and cannot afford to pay privately to get the help they need [4]). It is further argued, against the official view, that the belief that the development of new medicines and technologies must fuel growing patient demand *ad infinitum* is based on a myth [5]. It is argued that just as a doubling of public toilets or public bus services would not automatically double the desire (or need) of the public to make use of them, so too there is a finite amount of kidney disease, a limit to the number of people who can benefit from coronary by-pass surgery, and so on. Perhaps if more buses were supplied very cheaply, or even at no cost to the user at all, their use would increase, but even so there will always be a natural limit on the number of people who would like to travel from A to B at one time.

It is not easy to judge which one of these positions – the 'official line' or that of the 'rebel camp' – is correct. Clearly, both are at least partly true. For instance, where there are more potential recipients than donated organs there is an undeniable scarcity of this particular resource. On the other hand, it is equally incontrovertible that if money were to be taken from some expensive 'high-tech' or over-provided medical services, and spent instead on the provision of better and more comprehensive 'preventive services', many 'health needs' now not met because of scarcity could be provided for.

What is clearest of all though, is that there are considerable philosophical and practical uncertainties underlying the 'resources debate', most of which are unlikely to be resolved in the foreseeable future. The nature of 'health care cost' and 'health care benefit' is not agreed in theory [6]. Nor is it yet physically possible to collate even the simple financial costs of many modern health services [7]. And even if credible classifications and calculations were to be developed, even if someone were to invent a comprehensive 'health service slide rule', the accuracy and relevance of these taxonomies and methods of calculating would inevitably be challenged. It would, for instance, remain the case that different individuals would value even identical services (and identical results) in different ways. For one person a few more days of life, even in great pain, might be of immense value – while for another there would be no point at all.

7.12 Nursing in scarcity

What can nurses do when faced with such intangibles? These days almost all nurses work in environments where managers, and others, are openly concerned about efficiency, avoiding waste, and reducing cost wherever possible.

- What is the nurse, concerned about how best to use scarce resources, to do?
- How can she be fair?
- How can she deal with perceived injustice?
- How can she make any difference at all?

Whether or not any individual can make a difference within massive, complex systems depends on two factors. Firstly, and obviously, what she can do depends on whether or not she is in a position of any power and influence. Secondly, and less obviously, what she can do depends upon the clarity with which she has formulated her goals.

Philosophy (or clear thinking) can do nothing about the first factor, but it can help (albeit only a little) with the second. With practice a nurse can improve her understanding of both general situations and her own circumstances, she can learn to define the meaning of key terms (such as 'resource', 'rationing' and 'fairness'), and she can become better able to identify her role (and the limits of her role).

It is not possible, in the space of a short chapter, to provide a philosophical education. In order to learn philosophy there is no substitute for a carefully formulated programme of study undertaken, with expert guidance, over several years. However, it is possible to show how a philosophically informed nurse might at least begin to react to resource allocation problems, and in so doing to offer insight into one method of coping with seemingly impossible situations.

7.13 A number – or a free person?

Nursing is a hierarchical, and often authoritarian profession. All groups of nurses have 'pecking-orders', and those nurses who do not toe the line can, in some circumstances, suffer severe reprimand. This is a deep-seated aspect of nursing culture. It is an equally long-established tradition that most nurses are of a lower rank to doctors. These circumstances are changing somewhat nowadays, with the advent of nurse managers, and as nursing has come to be regarded as a profession in its own right. However, for very many nurses it remains the case that, in their working lives, they are able to exert only a very limited influence on health service policy.

So, when it comes to '**doing the right thing**', most nurses apparently have very little choice – the 'right thing' is defined by 'the system' in which they are a 'cog' or a 'number' and their only option is to implement it. The 'right thing', in other words, is handed down to them (this might be called '**doing the right thing 1**'). Of course, there is an alternative form of 'doing the right thing', which can be defined as a nurse taking that course of action which she has, after careful deliberation, deemed to be the best – whether or not this is the action recommended by the system – the 'right thing', in this form, is a matter of conscience and intelligent reflection (this might be called '**doing the right thing 2**').

How might the nurse 'do the right thing' in the two case studies offered by Robert Lee in the first part of this chapter?

7.13.1 *Case One*

Consider again the first case study of the nurse (N) on night duty in charge of a small hospital where R brings V, the victim of a hit-and-run accident, despite the sign at the gate advising that there is no accident and emergency unit there (section 7.7).

As far as '**doing the right thing 1**' is concerned, Robert Lee has already given part of a possible answer that 'in purely legal terms, N would be free to refuse treatment to V and urge R and V to present themselves at the nearest accident and emergency department.' Officially the hospital does not provide accident and emergency services, so there is no legal obligation on the nurse to do anything. Furthermore, if this hospital is cost-conscious, and if the management have made it clear that emergency cases are not to be treated, then to '**do the right thing 1**' the nurse *must* turn the potential patient away – and must do so whatever her feelings about it, and whatever help she might have been able to give. In such circumstances – since she would have 'done the right thing' – there would clearly be no sanction that 'the authorities' could take against the nurse.

However, in this case (as in all cases) the nurse might instead consider '**doing the right thing 2**' – that is, she might not simply follow the regulation course, but first take the trouble to analyse the situation for herself – and then act according to the result of her own reasoning. Of course, if she decides that she must advise V and R that she cannot help them, and that they must attend the nearest accident and emergency hospital, then the practical outcome will be the same. The nurse, however, will have thought more thoroughly than if she had merely obeyed the rules, and may well feel more confident (and more in charge) as a result. But how is she to carry out this analysis? How might she structure her thinking if she decides to '**do the right thing 2**'?

N does have the option to help the injured person, but if she does so she might well place herself at greater personal risk than if she were simply to turn V and R away. As stated in section 7.7, 'once N opts to render care and assistance to V, then a duty of care arises and the question then relates to the applicable standard of care. It is clear that liability may result from negligent treatment or advice rendered by N or any failure of communication in providing V with emergency treatment . . .' So what should she do? Clearly, '**doing the right thing 2**' is the more complicated – and potentially more fraught – option. What factors should the nurse take into account? How might she begin to think clearly about this case?

If she does decide to deliberate on the situation she must do so quickly, and under considerable emotional pressure – neither of which are conducive to clear reasoning. Given this, the nurse might find it helpful to organise her thinking under these three distinct headings: **context**, **outcomes** and **obligations**.

Context

Firstly, N must assess the risk. 'Risk', of course, is a general term which might be interpreted in several ways. The nurse might, for instance, think about

- the risk to the injured party (if he is not instantly helped how will he be affected?);
- the risk to her conscience (what if she begins to help and the patient dies – or what if she does not help and the patient dies?)
- the risk to her future career, and so on.

She must also, prior to any further deliberation, decide whether any intervention that she could make would do any good. If it will not, and if it is clearly better that V attends a working clinic, then obviously that is where he should go. If, on the other hand, she decides that she could give some help, she must also work out how *effective* she would be and how *certain* she is of her judgment about her effectiveness. Also – if there are other patients whom she might be helping instead of V – she must consider whether she should assist them before she turns her attention to V.

Outcomes

The context, in this case as in most cases which nurses have to deal with, is one of uncertainty. N simply does not know for sure what the outcome of any of her options will be. Because, of this it is very important that she reflects, in the abstract, on her *priorities*.

- Is she, for example, most concerned with the reputation of the hospital?
- Is she concerned for the safety of her other patients, who may be endangered if she devotes herself solely to the care of V?
- Or is her priority the injured person directly in front of her?

She may not, in a short space of time, be able to think through all the ramifications, but it will help her considerably if she feels she understands which of these possible goals are – in principle – the most important.

Obligations

Does she have any obligations or duties which override the *context* and the *practicalities*? Must she, for instance, as a 'caring professional' do all she can to help V, who is clearly suffering? This is for her to decide. However, as she thinks about this she must be aware that not only must she justify her decision to herself, but that she may also have to justify it to others. So, if she decides that she is obliged to intervene wherever she sees suffering she must also be able to say whether this is a *general obligation*, and is always incumbent on her, or whether there are factors (such as *context* and *outcome*) that may sometimes cancel out such a duty.

7.13.2 *Case Two*

Consider now the second case study set out in section 7.8 of W, the night duty charge nurse believing that the standard of care had dropped prior to a patient dying in distressing circumstances.

In this case, even more than the first, there are evidently two distinct 'right things to do'. '**To do the right thing 1**' in this case is either to do nothing because the *context* is so overwhelming (the nurse may know that similar staffing difficulties are being experienced across the country – how can her situation be made an exception?), or to pursue the matter through the 'official channels', as set out in section 7.8. However, since all the 'official channels' are themselves part of the system which allows (or is forced to allow) such a situation to arise, it is extremely unlikely that this course of action will bring about an improvement in the situation on the nurse's ward. '**To do the right thing 1**' would almost certainly mean that little would change.

If the nurse '**does the right thing 2**' it may be a different matter. Although she might in the end reach the same conclusions as generated by '**doing the right thing 1**', the nurse must first try to think as an individual uninfluenced by the system. What, she might ask, *ought* to be done in these circumstances?

The questions she must address are similar to those considered by N in Case One, and again might usefully be divided into the three categories. What are the risks? Will 'whistle-blowing' be effective? How important is the nurse's career? (There are well-known examples of nurses destroying their careers in the pursuit of causes they believe to be just.)

- Are the nurse's *obligations* to her patients paramount – or does she have wider duties (to her colleagues or to those future patients she might not be able to care for if she is suspended from work, or sacked)?

- In principle, what *outcomes* does she value most highly? Is her own happiness paramount? Or is it crucial that the patients on her ward get the best possible service? If the latter, does it matter that if she succeeds in getting what she wants for her ward, resources may be moved from other hard-pressed parts of the hospital – so decreasing the quality of service to other patients?

- Finally, if she decides that the *context* is unacceptable, and that something must be done to improve it, then '**doing the right thing 1**' may very well cease to be an option.

7.14 Principled solutions?

Some nurses may find it helpful to try to apply 'ethical principles' to resource allocation dilemmas. This approach has been widely recommended in recent years, and most texts on 'nursing ethics' contain sizeable sections on 'basic', 'ethical' or 'philosophical' principles [8]. A quartet of principles are regularly advocated, and it is likely that most nurses will at least have heard of them. They are: 'non-maleficence' (do not harm), 'beneficence' (do good), 'respect autonomy' (respect the patient's choice), and 'justice' [9]. (See also section 2.5.)

The attraction of this group of principles is that they seem to offer an uncomplicated structure within which to organize one's thoughts. Moreover, it seems possible to seize on just one of these principles in order to 'solve' a dilemma. If, for instance, a nurse feels that a doctor is not taking the wishes of a patient seriously she might describe this as 'unethical' behaviour purely because the doctor is not 'respecting autonomy' (so ignoring or overriding any alternative justifications the medic might have). Most nurses will have personal experience of cases in which this has happened – and might well consider it fair criticism – but it is very important not to confuse *the assertion of single principles* (however justifiable) with 'ethical analysis'. The latter is a much more complicated procedure which – if it is to be done at all properly – must involve reflection upon a range of 'ethical principles' together with the other considerations (*context, outcomes, obligations*) already mentioned in this section.

This is not to say that the use of the principles is unhelpful. The point is that any thoughtful ethical analysis is bound to place considerable intellectual demands on the health care analyst. In Case Two it might appear that the hub of the matter is a straightforward clash between the ideal of 'efficiency' and the principles of 'justice'. It might, in other words, seem to nurse W that her patients are being unjustly treated, and that their interests are regarded as secondary to those of the hospital as a whole (which must be run as 'efficiently' as possible). However, if W is seriously to argue this case then it is not enough for her merely to cry 'unjust!'.

'Justice' can be understood in more than one way, and can even be interpreted in ways which contradict each other. There are those who think that the key to understanding 'justice' is to treat people first and foremost in accord with what they *deserve*; others disagree – arguing that the basic criterion of justice is *need*; and there is a further group who believe that justice can come about only when peoples' *rights* are upheld [10]. What is more, sophisticated analysts tend to blend and adapt these different understandings in subtle ways, depending on the matter under scrutiny. Any contemplative analysis of the merits (or justice) of the management of the acutely ill patients must consider and explain what justice *means* in this case (whether the patients have the same *right* to treatment as other patients in the hospital – and so no special priority; whether they have *needs* of such gravity that they are entitled to treatment before those with lesser needs; whether this set of patients *deserves* priority treatment for some reason – whether they merit privileged attention).

Philosophers are used to such discussions, and often spend much time trying to disentangle the various issues, only to see them knot together again the moment they move their attention elsewhere. Such detailed reflection requires a fair amount of expertise – and countless hours – neither of which are usually available to the nurse. And this can place the nurse who sees that these are complex matters, and who recognizes that they can be properly dealt with only by careful analysis, at a considerable disadvantage. If she tries to protest in an intelligent way it is very easy to defeat her. Her opponent can say: 'We don't have the time for this sort of reflection'; or, 'What you are suggesting requires an analysis of *everything* we do, and this is not a practical proposition' (which of course means that everything can continue unchanged – inertia is not only a natural tendency but also a powerful weapon in the hands of those who are happy with the status quo). Her opponent might also ask: 'What do you mean by justice?', knowing full well that any credible answer must take more time and effort than almost any nurse can give (and knowing that even if the nurse does attempt an answer it will be very easy to say later: 'please spell out your interpretation of need/rights/equity' or whatever other terms she has not fully explained).

In such circumstances the nurse has three strategies open to her. She might spend many hours developing her case (she might even enlist the help of a trained philosopher); she might take a simpler course – and analyse her work problems using the '*context, outcomes* and *obligations*' framework (in the knowledge that this is by no means all there is to ethical analysis); or she might take her opponent on, on his own terms. Whenever he says, 'Could you expand on that?' or 'What do you mean?', then the nurse might ask in turn 'What do *you* mean by efficiency?', 'How do you justify removing resources from this ward and increasing them on that?' or 'What are your principles for resource allocation within this hospital, and on what grounds do you justify these?'

7.15 Conclusion

This part of the chapter has raised questions, but not attempted to answer them. That is for the individual nurse to decide, and there are many books and papers available to which she might turn for more detailed instruction. What is most important is that each nurse realizes the complexity of any resource problem she is facing, and, if she so decides, is able to tackle it in a systematic manner. If she genuinely tries to do this, and if she feels she has arrived at a defensible decision, then there is probably little more that she can do. She cannot change the world, and whatever she does she is hardly likely to unsettle governments focused so intently on financial balance sheets.

It may be, though, that a great deal rests on the following question, and how it is answered in the coming years: whether nurses in general continue '**to do the right thing 1**'; or whether the profession increasingly aims '**to do the right thing 2**' (and commits its own resources wholeheartedly to ensuring this). If the former, then it is hard to see how nurses will be able to justify their claim to professional status, but if the latter, and the majority of nurses become able and willing to think through the question 'How *best* might I act in this situation?' (rather than ask 'What am I *supposed* to do here?') then nurses, as a group, might perform an enormous service – they might open up the NHS to internal debate – to genuine conversation (without fear of sanction and reprisal) about how best to deliver public health services – and not least when there are not enough of them to go round.

7.16　Notes and references

1. See *Health Care Analysis* 1993; 1(1): *passim*.
2. Williams, A. 'Cost-Effectiveness Analysis: is it ethical?' *Journal of Medical Ethics*, 1992; 18: pp 7–11.
3. Harris, J. 'Unprincipled QALYs: a response to Cubbon' *Journal of Medical Ethics*, 1991; 17: pp 185–8.
4. Hackler, C. 'Health Care Reform in the United States', *Health Care Analysis*, 1993; 1(1): 5–13.
5. Smith, A. Qualms about QALYs. *The Lancet* 1987, 1134–36.
6. Seedhouse, D.F. *Fortress NHS: A Philosophical Review of the National Health Service.* Chichester: John Wiley and Sons, 1994.
7. Culyer, A. (1992) 'The Morality of Efficiency in Health Care – Some Uncomfortable Implications', *Health Economics*, 1992: 1(1): p 7–18.
8. Thompson, I. Melia, K.M., Boyd, K.M. *Nursing Ethics*, Edinburgh: Churchill Livingstone, 1988.
9. Gillon, R. *Philosophical Medical Ethics*, Chichester: John Wiley and Sons, 1985.
10. Miller, D. *Social Justice*, Oxford; Oxford University Press 1976.

Chapter 8
Mental Health Nursing

A The Legal Perspective
Michael Gunn

Of the many legal issues which face nurses working with people with mental illness or a learning disability, five will be considered in this chapter: treatment under the Mental Health Act 1983 [1]; treatment falling outside that Act; the use of the nurse's holding power under section 5(4) of the Mental Health Act 1983; the care and management of violent or aggressive patients; and the debate about the possibility of compulsory treatment in the community.

8.1 Treatment under the Mental Health Act 1983

Treatment for mental disorder may lawfully be given under the Mental Health Act 1983 provided the patient is detained under the Act under a non-emergency section. It is important to stress that treatment for physical problems is not under consideration here. If nurses are to be involved in the treatment of a patient, they must first be able to satisfy themselves whether the patient is detained under a relevant section. The fifth Biennial Report of the Mental Health Act Commission [2] has stressed the importance of the nurses' role, which the following addresses.

8.1.1 First stage: is the patient a detained patient?

A nurse must be able to make sure that the appropriate detention documentation for a non-emergency section is present in the patient's ward file. The nurse is, therefore, looking for documentation which indicates that the patient is detained under:

- section 2 (for assessment including medical treatment),
- section 3 (for treatment),
- section 36 (remand of accused person to hospital for treatment),
- section 37 (hospital order, with or without a restriction order under section 41),

- section 38 (an interim hospital order),
- section 46 (an order relating to a member of the armed forces),
- section 47 (a transfer of a prisoner, with or without restrictions under section 49), or
- section 48 (transfer of a civil or remand prisoner, with or without restrictions under section 49).

It is not necessary for the nurse to be sure that the patient is lawfully detained. The function of ascertaining the legality and appropriateness of detention is for the hospital managers, a function which is normally delegated to the medical records department. In any case, section 6(3) of the Mental Health Act 1983 ensures that it is appropriate to rely on the forms since it provides:

'Any application for the admission of a patient under this Part of this Act which appears to be duly made and to be founded on the necessary medical recommendations may be acted upon without further proof of the signature or qualification of the person by whom the application or any such medical recommendation is made or given or of any matter of fact or opinion stated in it.' [2a]

What is usually required, therefore, is that the nurse file, and then be able to find in the notes, the relevant forms indicating that the patient has been admitted under one of the sections to which reference has already been made. If the patient has been admitted under section 2, the nurse is looking for

(1) the application form which must be either Form 2 (where the nearest relative was the applicant) or Form 3 (where an approved social worker was the applicant),
(2) a form for the medical recommendation (either one copy of Form 4 where the recommendation was done jointly or two copies of Form 5 where the recommendations were done separately) and also
(3) Form 15 which indicates that the patient has been accepted by the hospital as a detained patient.

If the patient has been admitted under section 3, the nurse is similarly looking for

(1) the relevant application form (Form 8 where the applicant is the nearest relative and Form 9 where the applicant is an approved social worker),
(2) the relevant form stating the medical recommendations (one copy of Form 10 where there is a joint medical recommendation and

two copies of Form 11 where there are separate recommendations) and
(3) a copy of Form 15.

If the patient is detained under section 36, section 37, section 38, or
section 46 there must be documentation from a court indicating the
imposition of the section. If the patient is detained under section 47 or
section 48, there must be a warrant from the Home Secretary directing
the transfer of the patient to the hospital.

8.1.2 Second stage: does the treatment fall within the Mental Health Act?

Nurses must be able to satisfy themselves that the treatment proposed is
treatment which may lawfully be carried out under the Mental Health
Act 1983. Medical treatment is widely defined by the Act in section
145(1):

'"[M]edical treatment" includes nursing, and also includes care,
habilitation and rehabilitation under medical supervision . . .'

For the purposes of assessing the legality of the particular activity in
question, treatment is classified into three groups.

(1) Psychosurgery and surgical implantation of hormones
For psychosurgery or the surgical implantation of hormones to reduce
male sexual drive [3] to be performed, the patient's consent must be
verified by a second opinion approved doctor (appointed as such by the
Secretary of State for Health and known as a 'SOAD') and two members of the Mental Health Act Commission (from an internal panel
appointed for this purpose). These three must 'have certified in writing
that the patient is capable of understanding the nature, purpose and
likely effects of the treatment in question and has consented to it'
(section 57(2)(a)). Also the SOAD must certify that, 'having regard to the
likelihood of the treatment alleviating or preventing a deterioration of
the patient's condition, the treatment should be given' (section 57(2)(b)).
These requirements are certified as being satisfied by the completion of
Form 37. If there is no Form 37, the treatment cannot go ahead. Whilst
being treatments which raise considerable ethical and legal issues, these
two forms of treatment for mental disorder are carried out relatively
rarely [4] on detained patients, and attention is, therefore, concentrated
on the second group of treatments instead.

(2) Medicines and electro-convulsive therapy
The second group of treatments for mental disorder consists of electro-

convulsive therapy (ECT) and the continuation of the administration of medicine, by any means, for mental disorder [5] three months after the person first took a medicine when a detained patient. These are two very common treatment methods [6]. For nurses, it is essential that they ensure that their involvement is lawful. Numerous issues arise with regard to the administration of medicine. Nurses will either be involved in the distribution of medicines for self-administration or actually undertake the administration of the medicines. Once the first stage has been assessed, that is that the person is a detained patient, the nurse must know whether the administration of medicine requires the existence of a form. Unless three months have elapsed whilst the person has been a detained patient since the first administration of a medicine, there is no need for a form. This is because until the three month limit is reached the administration of medicine falls within the third group of treatments considered below. Once the three month rule applies, a form is necessary, because it records whether the Act is satisfied.

The three month rule causes some confusion, which is one reason why the Mental Health Act Code of Practice has been revised [7]. The Code now provides, at paragraph 16.11:

> '[The three month] period starts on the occasion when medication for mental disorder was first administered by any means during any period of continuous detention ... The medication does not necessarily have to be administered continuously throughout the three month period.'

If the nurse has ascertained that it is three months since the detained patient first had medicine for the mental disorder, the nurse must assess whether further medication may lawfully be provided. There are alternatives. Either the patient must have consented to it and that consent is verified by either the patient's own doctor (the responsible medical officer) or a SOAD, that is, they have 'certified in writing that the patient is capable of understanding [the] nature, purpose and likely effect [of the treatment] and has consented to it' (section 58(3)(a)). Or, if the patient either cannot or will not consent, the medication may continue if a SOAD has 'certified in writing that the patient is not capable of understanding the nature, purpose and likely effects of that treatment or has not consented to it but that, having regard to the likelihood of its alleviating or preventing a deterioration of [the patient's] condition, the treatment should be given' (section 58(3)(b)). The simplest way for the nurse to ensure that one of these alternatives has been satisfied, is by checking that the appropriate form is in existence. If the patient is consenting, the treatment must be covered by a Form 38; if the patient is not consenting, the treatment must be covered by a Form 39. For the nurse, the question is not so much whether the patient has consented or not, but whether there is a form apparently proper on its face which entitles the nurse to be involved in the treatment of the detained patient in question.

In most hospitals, where this matter has been given careful thought, a copy of the relevant form is kept with the medicine card, so that the legal authorization for the treatment of a detained patient may be checked every time a drug is administered. This is a simple procedure which enables an easy check to be made. It is surprising, however, how frequently the relevant form is not kept with the treatment card and how frequently the nurse does not realise the significance of the form or the importance of checking that it covers the treatment in question.

A number of other issues are raised. First, there is no statutory requirement for the review of treatment with consent as covered by a Form 38 [8]. The Mental Health Act Code of Practice, however, requires at paragraph 16.20 that it be reviewed at regular, though unspecified, intervals. Practice suggests that such reviews should take place at intervals of not longer than two years, although it is submitted that there are no real logistical problems with expecting review on an annual basis. If, therefore, a nurse is involved in the administration of medicine to a patient for whom a Form 38 is used, and that form covers the treatment but the form is more than two years old, it is suggested that the nurse ought to be raising questions about the necessity for review of the validity of the form. Review is expected not just because it is good practice to review treatment regimes, but also because it enables regular consideration to be given to the question of the patient's continued consent. Although a patient has the right to withdraw her or his consent [9], reliance on such action is inappropriate, and the treatment regime deserves reconsideration at fairly regular intervals. Further, if the doctor who originally signed the Form 38 is no longer the patient's responsible medical officer, there is a need for a new Form 38 [10].

Secondly, cases are often discovered in which the drug or its dosage listed on the Form 38 has changed since the form was originally signed. In that case the treatment may fall outside the law. In fact, there is no requirement that specific drugs be named, or specific dosages. Indeed, the Mental Health Act Code of Practice provides, at paragraph 16.12, that the doctor 'should indicate on the certificate the drugs proposed by the classes described in the British National Formulary (BNF), the method of their administration and the dose range (indicating the dosages if they are above BNF advisory limits)' [11]. However, where specific drugs are named, no further drug may be administered unless a new form is produced. Where a specific dosage is stated, no change in dosage level may be made, unless a new form is produced. This is why SOADs when signing Form 39s do not list specific drugs, but categories of drugs according to the BNF and do not specify dosages unless they are above the BNF recommended upper limits.

The following case study may illustrate the problems.

On one ward a patient was detained under section 3 of the Mental Health Act 1983, and that detention had been renewed under section 20 of the Act. The patient was taking drugs, and there was a Form 39 indicating that the patient was not capable of understanding the nature, purpose and likely effects of the drugs but that they should be given. On examination of the ward file, the original section papers were readily available, but their renewal, though in the file, was hidden away, as also was the Form 39. The nurse in question did not know the significance of either form and would not have been able to find either of them.

The treatment was lawful, the patient's detention was lawful, but the nurse was not in a position to indicate that authorization, and so was not protecting her legal position. This indicates a dangerous lack of knowledge, which admittedly is infrequent.

Little mention has been made of electro-convulsive therapy [12]. It is a treatment of some concern when it is used. Second opinions are usually provided, whether the treatment is ECT or medication. There are many possible reasons for this. They range from the sinister one of improper collusion between doctors to the more likely alternatives that most doctors recommend acceptable treatment for mental disorder or amendments to treatment plans are made after discussion between the responsible medical officer and the SOAD [13]. Indicators for the usage of ECT are well documented. Here is not the time to debate the rights and wrongs of this particular form of treatment, but it is worth repeating Fennell's point that the question is whether there are 'appropriate and effective safeguards' [14].

The nurse has a role not only in the administration of the treatment itself but also in the assessment of whether the treatment should take place. As with the administration of medicine, the patient may consent. If so, and if the nurse were concerned about the patient's ability to consent, it is a matter of some debate as to what then the nurse may do. If raising it with the consultant has no effect, suggesting that it would be sensible for a SOAD to be called in would be the best route to take. If, however, that is not done, recording dissent may be thought to be the most appropriate step for the nurse to take. This would then be picked up by the Mental Health Act Commission, which might wish to have the matter investigated. This approach, however, may place the nurse in a particularly difficult ethical position. It is always possible for electro-convulsive therapy to be authorized by a SOAD where the patient is consenting. A SOAD must be involved where the patient does not or will not consent.

(3) One of the four treatments in an emergency

Before passing on to the third group of treatments, it is necessary to note that the requirements listed for both of the first two groups of treatment may be side-stepped in an emergency. In these cases, it is important for nurses to ensure that they are satisfied that the criteria of section 62 are satisfied, since reliance upon another person's view (i.e. the doctor) may not be sufficient to protect the nurse from action where the treatment turns out to be unlawful. At the least, it is necessary for the nurse to ensure that there is documentation that section 62 has been satisfied. This may be done via a local form (as recommended in the Mental Health Act Code of Practice at para. 16.19) or some other recording system.

It may be necessary for the nurse to assess whether the treatment actually satisfies section 62. The section provides

'(1) Sections 57 and 58 above shall not apply to any treatment –
(a) which is immediately necessary to save the patient's life; or
(b) which (not being irreversible) is immediately necessary to prevent a serious deterioration of his condition; or
(c) which (not being irreversible or hazardous) is immediately necessary to alleviate serious suffering by the patient; or
(d) which (not being irreversible or hazardous) is immediately necessary and represents the minimum interference necessary to prevent the patient from behaving violently or being a danger to himself or others.'

and

'(3) For the purposes of this section treatment is irreversible if it has unfavourable physical or psychological consequences and hazardous if it entails significant physical hazard.'

Frequently, this section has caused debate. However, it should very rarely be used. It can only apply where the patient is detained and where one of the four forms of treatment, only, is proposed: that is psychosurgery, the surgical implantation of hormones to reduce male sexual drive, the administration of medicines after the first three months and electroconvulsive therapy [15]. This emergency section applies to *no* other form of treatment. It is difficult to see how psychosurgery or the surgical implantation of hormones can be carried out in an emergency. The latter treatment is almost unheard of in any case. Further, it is difficult to see how the requirements of the section can ever be satisfied with regard to the administration of medicines. Even if a patient has only once been administered a medicine for mental disorder, the three month rule operates at which point an assessment of that patient's need for medication, including prn (or as required) medication [16], should be made and depending upon that outcome, a Form 38 or Form 39 obtained. It is, therefore, the case that section 62 is only of any value with regard to the provision of ECT in an emergency, e.g. someone in a catatonic stupor who might otherwise die.

(4) All other forms of treatment for mental disorder

The third group is treatment for mental disorder given by or under the supervision of the patient's responsible medical officer. In these cases, section 63 provides that the patient's consent is not necessary. In some cases it is clear that the treatment is for the mental disorder from which the patient is suffering, for example, behaviour modification. In some cases it is clear that the treatment is not for the mental disorder from which the patient is suffering, for example, medication for pneumonia. But in some cases, it is not at all clear to decide.

The most recent controversial issue has been to consider the question of anorexia nervosa. Recent case law concerning young people has not considered this treatment under the Mental Health Act (*Re W* (1992)). It is the view of the Mental Health Act Commission, as expressed in its Fourth Biennial Report, that 'severe anorexia nervosa falls within the definition of mental disorder' [17]. In that case the person may be admitted to hospital, provided the other criteria are satisfied, under section 2 of the Mental Health Act 1983 for assessment (which may include medical treatment). It is also the view of the Mental Health Act Commission that 'treatment of anorexia nervosa necessary for the health or safety of the patient, including involuntary feeding and maintenance of hydration, is permissible in patients whose anorexia is causing serious concern' [18].

The only basis upon which this opinion may be predicated is that these forms of activity fall within the definition of treatment within the Act and that section 63 is the relevant section authorizing treatment. No-one, it is submitted, can dispute that, given the wide definition of medical treatment in the Act, involuntary feeding does fall within 'treatment'. Anorexia nervosa is a mental disorder, but the essential question, as required by the wording of section 63, is whether the treatment is *for* the mental disorder from which the patient is suffering. If it is for a consequence of the mental disorder or in order to keep the person alive in order to enable treatment for the mental disorder to be carried out, it is at least arguable that involuntary feeding cannot be treatment for mental disorder and therefore cannot be authorized under the Mental Health Act. It is submitted that the view of the Mental Health Act Commission may be relied upon by staff presented with these difficult issues, and this has been confirmed by recent case law [19].

No consideration has been given to the recent case law concerned with people under 18, because the law on which the decision was based, that a person with anorexia could be treated, is different when the law relating to adults is considered. The one exception to this general rule would be if the view were taken that the person suffering from anorexia was unable to consent to treatment, in which case involuntary feeding could be justified under the common law. This argument does not affect the propositions made concerning interpretation of the 1983 Act.

8.2 Treatment outside the Mental Health Act 1983

For the nurse, the questions are often fairly straightforward when the person is a detained patient and the treatment falls within the Act. However, the position is not so clear cut where the treatment falls outside the Act. The nurse may be involved with the care of a person who is an informal patient, who is a patient detained under an emergency section of the Act, or who is a patient for whom treatment for a physical disorder is proposed. In these cases, Part IV of the Mental Health Act is of no assistance.

8.2.1 *First stage: is the patient competent?*

If treatment is to be provided in these circumstances, it must be first ascertained whether the person is competent to consent to treatment. It is always to be presumed that patients are competent, whatever label they may carry or whatever history they may have. It is only if it is shown that the patient is not competent that anything other than the consent of the patient may be relied upon. Despite the clear importance of this requirement, it is surprising to discover that the matter had not been considered by the courts until it was peripherally considered by the Court of Appeal in *Re T* (1992) and centrally by the High Court in *Re C* (1994). The guidance these cases provide is at odds. The test propounded from *Re T* is simply that the person must understand in broad terms the nature of the proposed treatment. In *Re C* (1994) the court adopted a test requiring that the patient must 'sufficiently understand the nature, purpose and likely effects of the proffered' treatment. In so saying, the judge adopted a proposal by an expert witness that the decision-making process should be divided into three stages: 'first, comprehending and retaining treatment information, second, believing it and, third, weighing it in the balance to arrive at choice.'

Otherwise, the guidance that exists, and which is likely to be followed in view of its source, is to be found in the Mental Health Act Code of Practice [20] which provides: at paragraph 15.10:

'An individual in order to have capacity must be able to:
- understand what medical treatment is and that somebody has said that he need it and why the treatment is being proposed;
- understand in broad terms the nature of the proposed treatment;

- understand the principal benefits and risks;
- understand what will be the consequences of not receiving the proposed treatment;
- possess the capacity to make a choice.

It must be remembered:

- any assessment as to an individual's capacity has to be made in relation to a particular treatment proposal;
- capacity in an individual with a mental disorder can be variable over time and should be assessed at the time the treatment is proposed;
- all assessments of an individual's capacity should be fully recorded in the patient's medical notes.'

and further at paragraph 15.11:

'The fact that a person is suffering from a mental disorder does not mean that he is thereby incapable of giving consent. Capacity to consent is variable in people with mental disorder; not everyone is equally capable of understanding the same explanation of a treatment plan. A person is more likely to be able to give valid consent if the explanation is appropriate to the level of his assessed ability. This does not necessarily mean that an individual should be given less information. Thus, the capacity to consent should be assessed in relation to the particular patient, at the particular time, as regards the particular treatment proposed.'

The nurse's involvement may be either to assist in an assessment of a person's competence to make a treatment decision or to decide whether there is sufficiently clear guidance available to act on the basis that the person is not competent. In the first scenario, nurses are being asked to proffer independent views from their professional perspective on the matters raised by the definition of competence just quoted. In the second scenario, nurses need to be sure that there is an indication that the person is incompetent so that the treatment in which they are to engage is justified without the patient's consent. It should not always involve the nurse in requesting an assessment of competency, although there will be cases where that is required, but should involve the nurse in being able to check the records to see whether the patient is regarded at the time of the treatment as being not competent to consent to the particular treatment in question. To be involved in these various activities, therefore, the nurse needs to be professionally qualified and skilled to assist in determinations of competency, needs to be aware of the various approaches and to be capable of identifying the warning signs that the patient may not be competent to consent. The nurse also needs to be sufficiently aware to consider the legal situation prior to being involved in the treatment of the patient.

8.2.2 Second stage: where the patient is competent

It is quite clear that, where patients are competent, their decisions must be followed. This is so even where the patient is dying and it is life-saving treatment which is refused. So, in *Re T* (1992), the Court of Appeal accepted the principle that an adult may refuse life-saving treatment, (although it was decided, on the facts of the particular case, that the adult woman in question had been subject to undue influence in refusing her consent). Although there are many legal issues arising in this area, particularly about the obligation to provide information, these have been covered in detail in Chapter 6 and other issues relating to mental health patients demand consideration.

The only possible exception to this was discovered in a highly controversial case, *Re S* (1992) where a judge authorized a caesarean section on a woman who had refused because it was contrary to her religious views. It should be noted that the judgment was made under extreme pressure of time as the woman (who was not represented) was already in difficulties in labour.

8.2.3 Third stage: where the patient is not competent

If a patient is not competent, treatment may be given provided it is in her best interests, in the sense that a responsible body of other similar treatment providers would also give the same treatment, as was decided by the House of Lords in F v. *West Berkshire Health Authority* (1989). In some cases, the treatment provider will have sought the assistance of the courts in determining whether the treatment is in the patient's best interests. This should happen in any case where sterilization of an adult not competent to consent is being contemplated [21]. It is submitted that it should also happen in all cases where the proposed treatment is ethically or morally more complicated than the usual forms of treatment. This submission would extend to a proposal for termination of pregnancy even though a court, in *Re SG* (1991), decided that a declaration was not necessary where the criteria of the Abortion Act 1967 were satisfied. However, these criteria do not address the question of whether the procedure is in the best interests of the woman in question [22].

Whoever is the treatment provider must ascertain whether, according to the standards of their profession, the treatment which is proposed would be carried out by a responsible body of that profession. The question which will arise is whether the nurse is required to comply with the doctor's request that treatment be provided. This places nurses in a difficult position where they are not satisfied that the treatment being proposed is indeed in the best interests of the patient according to proper nursing standards. In a case such as this, which is more fully considered elsewhere in this book, it is submitted that the nurse must be very wary of simply following the doctor's instructions without at least raising and recording any doubts there may be about the proposed course of action.

A best interests approach is not a surprising one where the patient is not and has not been capable of expressing any treatment wishes. But defining a person's best interests may be problematic and fail adequately to achieve the proper balance, as Fennell points out, between the obligation to show respect for persons (that is concern for the person's welfare) and the obligation to respect the wishes of the person – that is the balance between paternalism and autonomy [23]. At this stage it should be noted that the nature of the best interests test is that it does not solve the 'ethical differences which may occur within care teams concerned with the treatment of incapable patients' [24].

8.2.4 *Looking to the future: the work of the law commission*

Clarity and precision are lacking in the current legal position where treatment is being considered for a person who cannot consent. If the proposals to be found in the Law Commission's Consultation Document, *Mentally Incapacitated Adults and Decision-Making: Medical Treatment and Research* [25], are introduced then clarity and precision will be provided. These proposals would be welcome not merely because they would offer certainty, but also because they are based upon a statement of principles which the Commission has explicitly made [26]:

'(i) that people should be enabled and encouraged to take for themselves those decisions which they are able to take;
(ii) that where it is necessary in their own interests or for the protection of others that someone else should take decisions on their behalf, the intervention should be as limited as possible and concerned to achieve what the person himself would have wanted; and
(iii) that proper safeguards should be provided against exploitation, neglect, and physical, sexual or psychological abuse.'

Medical treatment
The Commission, therefore, makes proposals for consultation which are intended to offer 'limited intervention [so] that any substitute decisions should be taken at the lowest appropriate level and with the least possible procedural formality [27].' On the basis of this approach, the Law Commission makes proposals in this the second in a series of

consultation documents concerned with ' "medical treatment" . . . used in a wide sense to include surgical, medical or dental treatment, any procedure undertaken for the purpose of diagnosis, and any procedure (including the administration of an anaesthetic) which is ancillary to such treatment. As in the Mental Health Act 1983 the expression also includes nursing, and care, habilitation and rehabilitation under medical supervision [28].'

Incapacity

In summary, the proposals involve first a definition of incapacity. There would be three different routes to a finding of incapacity [29]:

(1) that the person should be suffering from a mental disorder as defined in section 1 of the Mental Health Act 1983; and 'should be considered unable to take the medical treatment decision in question if he or she is unable to understand an explanation in broad terms and simple language of the basic information relevant to taking it, including information about the reasonably foreseeable consequences of taking or failing to take it, or is unable to retain the information for long enough to take an effective decision.'

(2) that the person should be suffering from a mental disorder and although possessing the capacity to understand he or she 'is unable because of mental disorder to make a true choice in relation to it.'

(3) that the person whether or not suffering from a mental disorder is 'unable to communicate the decision in question to others who have made reasonable efforts to understand it.'

It is submitted that the first definition is an appropriate one. It is not sufficient to have a finding of mental disorder, including both mental illness and learning disability, but the presence of such a disorder is a precondition to a finding of incapacity. Since most incapacity is tied in somehow to a mental disorder this approach makes sense, without involving any necessary extra stigma, since there is no presumption made that a person with a mental disorder is incapable of consenting to treatment. The definition then relies upon a functional approach, which is the only sensible, workable and meaningful approach that can be taken to decision-making. There is, however, no explicit presumption of capacity stated in the proposals, although that is the current and indeed proper stance of the common law and is not to be departed from.

The second definition may resolve the problem of, for example, the intelligent person who has no difficulty in understanding information, but who cannot act upon it in the exercise of choice because of, for example, a delusional or obsessive belief.

The third definition, it is submitted, is highly controversial and subject to real potentiality for abuse. If this is to be accepted, guidelines to avoid lack of care in attempting to understand the person would have to be drawn up, because the vast majority of people are capable of communicating a decision, even if the person to whom it is communicated has great difficulty in understanding it.

Position where there is no anticipatory decision and an incompetent adult: a new statutory authority

The Commission allows for the recognition of anticipatory decisions made by the person whilst competent and for decisions made by a medical treatment attorney. If there is no anticipatory decision, the Commission proposes [30] that a 'treatment provider should be given a statutory authority ... to carry out treatment which is reasonable in all the circumstances to safeguard and promote the best interests of an incapacitated person or a person whom he or she has reasonable grounds for believing to be incapacitated.'

In deciding whether the treatment is in the best interests of the incapacitated person, the Commission proposes [31] that 'consideration should be given to

(1) the ascertainable past and present wishes and feelings (considered in the light of his or her understanding at the time) of the incapacitated person;
(2) whether there is an alternative to the proposed treatment, and in particular whether there is an alternative which is more conservative or which is less intrusive or restrictive;
(3) the factors which the incapacitated person might be expected to consider if able to do so, including the likely effect of the treatment on the person's life expectancy, health, happiness, freedom and dignity.'

It is difficult to see how the Commission could have avoided a best interests approach when there is no anticipatory decision. This approach gives priority to what the person would have decided if that is discernible, otherwise it provides objective criteria about which a body of general expertise may develop.

The Commission further proposes [32] that a 'treatment provider should be under a duty to consult the incapacitated person's "nearest relative" ... as far as is reasonably practicable ... and to have regard to the views of that person.'

A judicial forum for difficult cases

The Commission recognises that not all treatment questions can be resolved in the manner indicated, that is without the need to have recourse to a more formal decision-making process. The desire to keep things informal, though, is heartily to be welcomed. But, for use in some cases, the Commission proposes [33] that there be 'a judicial forum with a statutory jurisdiction:

(1) to make orders approving or disapproving the medical treatment of incapacitated patients; and
(2) to make declarations as to the patient's capacity or the scope or validity of the patient's own decisions.'

There is, therefore, a clear decision-making process.

In arriving at a decision the 'judicial forum must be satisfied that the making of an order will bring greater benefit to the incapacitated person than making no order at all [34].' The making of unnecessary orders should, therefore, be avoided and the forum will be required always to question itself as to the appropriateness of its involvement.

In making an order the forum will have to take into account specified criteria, which will ensure that the decisions made are appropriate to the scheme proposed by the Law Commission and will require the forum to adopt an appropriate, consistent and coherent approach to the cases that come before it. The forum will be required [35] to take into account:

'(1) the ascertainable past and present wishes and feelings (con-sidered in the light of his or her understanding at the time) of the incapacitated person;
(2) whether there is an alternative to the proposed treatment, and in particular whether there is an alternative which is more con-servative or which is less intrusive or restrictive;
(3) the factors which the incapacitated person might be expected to consider if able to do so, including the likely effect of the treat-ment on the person's life expectancy, health, happiness, free-dom and dignity, but not the interests of other people except to the extent that they have bearing on the incapacitated person's individual interests.'

The judicial forum will be able [36] to 'make an order giving or withholding approval to the giving, withholding or withdrawal of parti-cular medical treatment in respect of an incapacitated person.' Further, the forum will be able [37] to make recommendations rather than orders. It will also be able [38] to make a declaration that the person in question 'is not incapacitated, either in general or in relation to a par-ticular matter.' If a single issue order is not to be sufficient, the forum 'may appoint any suitable person who agrees to discharge the duties of a medical treatment proxy for that person. The proxy will have such powers in relation to that person's medical treatment as are specified in the order making the appointment' [39]. The medical proxy is to act in accordance with the same principles as the forum.

The Law Commission has taken great care [40] to ensure that guidance is offered with respect to matters concerning the work of a proxy which would otherwise have given rise to considerable controversy, so the proxy would be able to recover the expenses of acting, would be able to apply on behalf of the incapacitated person for access to records, would have 'no authority to refuse pain relief or "basic care", including nursing care and spoon-feeding', would have no authority to consent to treatment contrary to a valid anticipatory decision or to the taking of a step requiring the approval of the judicial forum or to which the incapacitated person objects. The Law Commission proposes [41] a clear application procedure to set in motion the role of the judicial forum.

Independent supervision of special category treatments
It is particularly welcome that the Law Commission proposes [42] to establish a special category of treatments which would require the 'approval of the judicial forum before they are taken in relation to an incapacitated person, except where the step is essential to prevent an immediate risk of serious harm to that person.' The special category would be subject to change, but the Law Commission identified [43] the following treatments to place within it:

- sterilization
- donation of non-regenerative tissue or bone marrow
- the withdrawal of life-necessitating nutrition or hydration.

The Law Commission invites views upon whether abortion and medical research should be included in the category. It is submitted that both should be included. Even though abortions may arise in an emergency, it must often be the case that a judicial forum hearing would be possible rather than merely relying upon the decision of the two doctors under the Abortion Act 1967.

It is, frankly, difficult to have any other view than admiration for the work of the Law Commission. Whilst people may not agree with some of the fine details, the overall structure is one clearly to be commended. It appears to satisfy the principles explicitly set by the Commission. The only real concern is whether it is feasible in the sense of being able to obtain governmental support when it contains significant resourcing issues. It is submitted that no workable solution can avoid increasing expenditure, and that this must be accepted as a consequence of dealing properly with the position of people not capable of making decisions for themselves. To avoid spending money would let down the clients and the staff.

8.3 The nurse's holding power - section 5(4) of the Mental Health Act 1983

The 1983 Act provided nurses with a specific power to detain patients for a short period of time [44], Section 5(4) provides:

'If, in the case of a patient who is receiving treatment for mental disorder as an in-patient in a hospital, it appears to a nurse of the prescribed class [45] –
(a) that the patient is suffering from mental disorder to such a degree that it is necessary for him to be immediately restrained from leaving the hospital; and
(b) that it is not practicable to secure the immediate attendance of a [doctor] for the purpose of furnishing a report under [section 5(2)], the nurse may record that fact in writing; and in that event the patient may be detained in the hospital for a period of six hours from the time when that fact is so recorded or until the earlier arrival at the place where the patient is detained of a [doctor] having power to furnish a report under [section 5(2)].'

This power presents a nurse who has appropriate training with an important professional responsibility. It is to be exercised by the nurse making a proper professional judgment as to whether the power should be exercised or, as the Mental Health Act Code of Practice puts it, at paragraph 9.1, '[i]t is the personal decision of the nurse and he [sic] cannot be instructed to exercise the power by anyone else.' If it is not exercised and the patient either comes to harm or harms someone else, it does not follow that the nurse is necessarily liable to any legal action. It must be assessed whether or not the decision not to exercise the power was taken reasonably. If it was a reasonable decision, that is it was a decision which a group of responsible qualified nurses would also have made in the circumstances, then no liability follows. It is a power in which there is an element of risk-taking and following sound guidance reduces without eliminating the risks.

The guidance of the Mental Health Act Code of Practice is to be found in paragraph 9.2:

'Before using the power the nurse should assess:
(a) the likely arrival time of the doctor as against the likely intention of the patient to leave. Most patients who express a wish to leave hospital can be persuaded to wait until a doctor arrives to discuss it further. Where this is not possible the nurse must try to predict the impact of any delay upon the patient;
(b) the consequences of a patient leaving hospital immediately – the

harm that might occur to the patient or others – taking into account:

- what the patient says he will do;
- the likelihood of the patient committing suicide;
- the patient's current behaviour and in particular any changes in usual behaviour;
- the likelihood of the patient behaving in a violent manner;
- any recently received messages from relatives or friends;
- any recent disturbance on the ward (which may or may not involve the patient);
- any relevant involvement of other patients.

(c) the patient's known unpredictability and any other relevant information from other members of the multi-disciplinary team.'

As the power is written, it appears that a form must be filled in prior to the act of restraint. In some cases this would be wholly impracticable, for example, where the patient unexpectedly leaps out of bed and runs out of the ward, it would be impracticable to fill in a form and then restrain the patient. Until recently, a simple and straightforward answer would have been given, which was that in those instances it would be proper to prevent the patient from leaving immediately and that a form should be filled in straight away. The legality for this action would have been found in the common law on one of a number of bases, such as prevention of crime, defence of others or the duty of care owed to the patient and the people living in the locality. Indeed, whilst the Mental Health Act Code of Practice does not directly deal with this question, paragraph 9.3, dealing with acute emergencies, could be read as a least implicitly lending support to this approach.

However, a House of Lords case has cast some doubt on this approach. In a Scottish case, *Black* v. *Forsey* (1988), the House decided that, in the context of the specific Scottish legislation, the common law power to 'arrest the insane' [46] could not be used where there was legislation dealing with the matter, but which could not be applied because of a specific statutory limitation. This would suggest that a trained nurse could not use the common law power but that an untrained nurse could. It is submitted that it is still correct to detain the patient before the documentation is completed and that this is justifiable either because it is not covered by the Scottish case or because the power being used is the common law power to prevent crime or defend other people, the exercise of which is not limited by the Scottish case.

Clearly, section 5(4) is a power which assumes an appropriate level of staffing. Indeed, paragraph 9.10 of the Mental Health Act Code of Practice states that '[a] suitably qualified nurse should be on all wards where there is a possibility of Section 5(4) being invoked.' Not only does appropriate staffing lessen the likelihood of the power being necessary; it is also an essential prerequisite for its use. If there are too few professionally qualified nurses on duty, the section cannot be exercised or can only be exercised with great difficulty. It is submitted that it is implicit in the Act, that a ward will be staffed by at least one nurse who is appropriately qualified. Many wards and/or hospitals will fail to realise this standard. If so, it is possible in the light of *Black* v. *Forsey*, though unlikely, that the patient could not legally be detained.

The Code of Practice appears to accept a different approach at paragraph 9.10. It provides that it is the responsibility of local management to assess those wards, in addition to the obvious, where it is possible that section 5(4) might be used, in which case 'they should ensure that suitable arrangements are in place for a suitably qualified nurse to be available should the power need to be invoked.' This implies that a nurse not working on the ward, perhaps not even having personal knowledge of the patient, may be brought in to exercise the section 5(4) power. It is questionable whether this is correct in the light of what section 5(4) provides.

In auditing the use of section 5(4), a question which must be asked is whether the section is being over-used. It must be stressed that there is no proper level of usage. If usage of section 5(4) is high, the question to be considered is whether more patients should be detained under the Act than is currently the case. If usage is low, it may be because there are a lot of detained patients or because methods of preventing patients leaving as alternatives to the section 5(4) power are used. In either case there would be interesting debates. In the first place whether sectioning was being used too frequently. In the second case, whether legally dubious methods of *de facto* detention are being used. It is when this sort of question is asked that significant controversies arise. Here one central issue is how frequently sectioning under the Act should be used.

8.3.1 Use of sectioning generally

In favour of greater use of the Act are the factors which indicate that the patient's legal position is formally protected under the Act. This protection will include some or all of the following:

- the requirements laid down in the Act for initial admission to a section,
- the requirements for renewal of detention where permissible,
- the right of application to a Mental Health Review Tribunal which has the power to discharge a patient,
- the provisions relating to consent to treatment, and
- the existence and powers of the Mental Health Act Commission.

If these provisions work well, no patient should be illegally or improperly detained in hospital, treatment should be provided only when it is right so to do, and the patient need not be proactive in raising issues. On the other hand, the detained patient's freedom of action is considerably curtailed by the very nature of detention.

In favour of informal admission is the reliance on the patient's decision-making which it entails thereby enhancing that individual's control over his or her life. But this does rely upon the ability to make decisions and take responsibility for those decisions. If people lack that capacity, their protection is greater under the Act as, detained patients unless and until a new jurisdiction is created which demands a reassessment of this perspective. Staff protection is also often greater where someone is detained under the Act rather than present in hospital informally.

8.3.2 *The wandering patient*

The other major controversy is over the use of methods, such as the confusion locks on doors, which mean that informal patients cannot leave the hospital but there is no exercise of statutory authority. The extent of the controversy can be realized by positing the case of the wandering patient. It is difficult for many staff to conceive that detention under the Act has a role to play in the case of an elderly confused patient who has a tendency to wander and thus be a hazard to self or others on the roads. Sectioning seems to be too dramatic a step to take. This is a view which deserves to be considered carefully but, first, it is to be noted that the possibility of locking wards is accepted in practice. Paragraph 18.27 of the Code of Practice states:

> 'The safety of informal patients, who would be at risk of harm if they were allowed to wander out of a ward or nursing home at will, can usually be secured by means of adequate staff and good surveillance. Combination locks and double handed doors to prevent mentally frail elderly people or people with learning disabilities (mental handicap) from wandering out should be used as little as possible and only in units where there is a regular and significant risk of patients wandering off accidentally and, as a result, being at risk of harm. There should be clear unit policies on the use of locks and other devices and a mechanism for reviewing decisions. Every patient should have an individual care plan which states explicitly why and when he will be prevented from leaving the ward. Patients who are not deliberately trying to leave the ward, but who may wander out accidentally may legitimately be deterred from leaving the ward by those devices. In the case of patients who persistently and purposely attempt to leave a ward or nursing home, whether or not they understand the risk involved, consideration must be given to assessing whether they

should be more appropriately detained in the hospital or a registered mental nursing home formally under the Mental Health Act rather than remain as informal patients.'

The extent to which this advice falls within the existing law is a matter of debate. Restricting a person's freedom is false imprisonment, but certain restrictions are permissible. Since the patients in these instances are owed a duty of care by the staff, it may be appropriate to determine that there is no false imprisonment where the patient is unthinkingly trying to leave, but that where the patient is making a purposeful desire to leave the ward prevention without statutory authority may be not lawful. Needless to say current guidance would suggest observance of the Code of Practice.

The other controversial aspect of this case is whether detention under the Act is necessarily inappropriate. To an extent this point has already been addressed by drawing attention, briefly, to the advantages for the patient of detention under the Act. It should also be noted that the staff have significant advantages in terms of the legal authority for their acts. However, against this must be set the philosophy that interferences in people's freedom of action should be entertained only where absolutely necessary. Whilst the Mental Health Act clearly engenders a variant of a paternalistic approach, it must be kept within bounds.

8.4 The management of violent or aggressive patients

For some considerable time patients who present violently or aggressively have been a matter of concern for the staff most closely involved with their care and treatment. As long ago as 1977, the Confederation of Health Service Employees in its report, *The Management of Violent or Potentially Violent Patients* [47], attempted to address this thorny matter.

8.4.1 *Common law justifications*

It is submitted that reliance upon the common law indicating that people may defend themselves or others is the proper basis upon which to authorize activity to deal with a violent or aggressive patient whether that be physical force, seclusion or medication. Where some sort of physical response is necessary, the least force necessary safely to contain the problem which the patient presents should be used. In many cases this may be holding the patient or properly trained staff using control and restraint techniques. Where such force is unlikely to be sufficient or where its use may be harmful to the patient, staff and/or other patients, seclusion may be necessitated. In some cases an appropriate alternative might be medication.

These activities have not been justified upon the basis that they are 'medical treatment' within the Act (where the person is a detained patient) or part of a treatment programme to which the patient has consented (where the person is an informal patient). Where the person is a detained patient, it is submitted that regarding these activities as 'treatment' in the light of the very wide definition of treatment, as is the case in the Mental Health Act Code of Practice (paragraph 18.15), is not correct. However wide the definition of treatment, it is still intended to have some curative or ameliorative purpose or expectation, which is not the case with the techniques under consideration. (Were the techniques under consideration those of behaviour modification, including time-out, the debate would be a different one. [48]) As regards informal patients since it is clear that they could refuse consent at any stage (which might lead to sectioning), it is difficult, though not impossible, to rely upon consent to treatment or consent to restraint as a justification.

The difficulties here presented are avoided by reliance upon self-defence as justifying the activities of the staff in restraining in some fashion a violent or aggressive patient.

8.4.2 *Seclusion*

It is assumed that seclusion, though controversial, is lawful and will continue to be used even if only rarely. 'Seclusion is the supervised confinement of a patient alone in a room which may be locked for the protection of others from significant harm' [49]. There is nothing inherent in seclusion which makes it unlawful. It is not controlled by statute. If abused, however, it is a response to challenging behaviour which unacceptably interferes with a patient's freedom of movement and, possibly, bodily integrity. It can be used for too long and can be used as a punishment rather than as an appropriate response to an incident of threatening behaviour. It can also result in the patient suffering harm whilst in seclusion.

It was because of the excesses frequently documented that the inquiry team at Ashworth recommended [50] that the technique be abolished. However, whilst it is laudable to argue for and expect a reduction in its use, it is not easy to see how seclusion can be abolished, even though many hospitals claim to have discontinued its use. Whilst patients presenting challenging behaviour may often be nursed so that no further action need be taken, it is submitted that there are some instances when further action is necessitated. In view of the time restraint on prolonged use of control and restraint and the inherent problems in using medication, it is hard to avoid the conclusion that separating someone from the company of others in a secure and safe environment can be a sensible and appropriate option.

It is essential that seclusion be properly used. The Mental Health Act

Code of Practice offers sound advice. Paragraph 18.17 provides that seclusion may be imposed by the nurse in charge of the ward, in addition to other people not likely to be available on the ward at the time. It is most likely that it is the ward nurse who will have to make the decision. Indeed, if it is possible to contact someone else, such as a doctor or a nursing officer, it may be that seclusion is inappropriate. Once a patient has been placed in seclusion, the duty of care owed by the staff to the patient demands that account be taken of the new circumstances, thus the Code further provides:

'18.18 A nurse should be readily available within sight and sound of the seclusion room at all times throughout the period of the patient's seclusion, and present at all times with a patient who has been sedated.

18.19 The aim of observation is to ascertain the state of the patient and whether seclusion can be terminated. The level should be decided on an individual basis, but a documented report must be made every 15 minutes.

18.20 *If seclusion needs to continue* a review should take place every 2 hours, carried out by 2 nurses in the seclusion room, and every 4 hours by a doctor. If seclusion continues for more than 8 hours consecutively or for more than 12 hours intermittently over a period of 48 hours, an independent review must take place with a consultant or other doctor of suitable seniority, a team of nurses and other health care professionals who were not directly involved in the care for the patient at the time the incident which led to the seclusion took place. If there is no agreement on ensuing action the matter should be referred to the unit general manager.'

The Code specifies the conditions of seclusion:

'18.21 Seclusion should be in a safe, secure and properly identified room, where the patient cannot harm himself, accidentally or intentionally. The room should have adequate heating, lighting, ventilation and seating. It is a matter for local judgement what the patient is allowed to take into the room, but he should always be clothed.

18.22 The room should offer complete observation from the outside, while also affording the patient privacy from other patients.'

8.5 The debate about compulsory treatment in the community

With the move towards closure of the large psychiatric hospitals, greater challenges are presented to those working with people with mental illness or learning disability. One particular challenge is that of treatment in the community. The case of Ben Silcock has graphically presented the issues. Here was a man suffering from schizophrenia who did not take his medication whilst living in the community who, therefore, became more and more ill, until he climbed into the lions' den at London Zoo.

The Mental Health Act proffers no direct solution since it does not provide for community treatment. It is possible for treatment to be continued under the provisions of Part IV of the Act whilst a detained patient is on leave in the community. But leave of absence can only last for a maximum of six months, at the end of which period patients must either be recalled and kept in hospital or be discharged (*R* v. *Hallstrom, ex parte W R* v. *Gardner, ex parte L* (1986) [51]. In consequence, there has been a long running debate about the advisability of a community treatment order. The latest phase has been the Report of an Internal Review by the Department of Health [52] which examined the issue in the wake of Silcock's case and in the light of the recent proposals of the Royal College of Psychiatrists for a Community Supervision Order [53].

The Internal Review recognized that there is a problem of sufficient magnitude to demand a response. They estimated, on the basis of a survey carried out by Dr Tom Burns of St George's Medical School, that 'there could be a national total of some 3,000 current patients in England and Wales whose RMOs [responsible medical officers] would consider them suitable for some form of community supervision provision [54].'

8.5.1 *More effective use of existing powers*

The Internal Review Team identified a number of responses. First, it recommended that existing powers be used more effectively. Most notably, attention is drawn [55] to the amendments to the Mental Health Act Code of Practice, paragraph 2.6 which attempts to make quite clear that sections 2 and 3 of the Mental Health Act 1983 may be used for the health of the patient *or* for the safety of the patient *or* for the protection of the others. The Mental Health Act may, therefore, be used in many instances where the potential patient presents no danger to others. It is entirely possible that professionals have been wary of using the Act as early as they are clearly entitled to. The Report also draws attention [56] to the possibility that guardianship might be used more frequently, although it is not a power which guarantees that the person under guardianship will receive treatment.

8.5.2 *Amendment to existing powers*

As already noted, leave of absence may enable treatment to be given in the community for a six month period. The Report recommends [57] that section 17 of the Mental Health Act be amended so as to allow leave of absence to be granted for a twelve month period. Such a recommendation involves no other change in the Act. The Report suggests [58] that this could only be an interim measure.

8.5.3 *Creation of a new power*

The Report recommends that a new response is required in the form of a new power. The Report does not recommend adoption of the proposal of the Royal College of Psychiatrists for a Community Supervision Order, but proposes the creation of a 'supervised discharge arrangement' [58a]. The main elements would be:

'(a) **Criteria**. The RMO is satisfied in the light of the patient's history, and after consulting others involved in his or her care, that there would be a serious risk to the health or safety of the patient or the safety of other people, or of the patient being exploited by other people, unless care was supervised.

(b) **Nature of conditions**. As well as embodying the principles of the care programme approach these should also include key features of guardianship. Thus:
- there should be a named key worker;
- there should be a clear treatment plan negotiated with the patient;
- the patient could be required to reside at a specified place;
- the patient could be required to attend for 'medical treatment, occupation, education or training';
- the key worker and other named staff involved in the patient's care would be entitled to have access to him or her.

Those involved in providing care should also have the power to convey the patient to a place he or she was to attend for treatment etc.

(c) **Procedure**. The conditions should be agreed with the key worker and any other agencies and people (including relatives) involved in the patient's care. Those drawing up the conditions would be responsible for ascertaining the patient's wishes and ensuring that they were taken into account as far as practicable.

(d) **Duration**. This could be based on the periods laid down at present for detention under section 3 – that is, six months initially, followed by a further six months, followed by periods of a year at a time. We see no particular reason to provide an overall time-limit, given the other safeguards we propose.

(e) **Failure to comply**. If the patient did not comply with the conditions, the key worker would, in consultation with the RMO and other members of the care team, institute an immediate review to establish what had gone wrong and propose any necessary changes to the plan.

(f) **Recall to hospital**. In the review, specific consideration would be given to whether the patient's condition had deteriorated so far as to meet the criteria for compulsory admission under the Act. If admission were found to be necessary, the arrangements for effecting this would be the responsibility of the RMO and the approved social worker concerned.

(g) **Patient's rights**. When supervised discharge was being proposed it would be open to the patient to apply to an MHRT (Mental Health Review Tribunal) for discharge without supervision. Thereafter, the patient should have a right to a tribunal hearing in each period of supervision, and automatic referral to a tribunal after three years if he or she had not applied sooner (in line with the existing arrangements for those detained under section 3)' [59].

8.5.4 *Assessing the proposals*

Is a new power necessary?

It is important to assess whether the case for a new power has been made out. The Report indicates that a survey has been undertaken, as reported earlier, which underpins the anecdotal evidence in favour and the evidence of a number of highly publicised incidents caused by people in the community not having received their treatment. The cynic would point out that it is the RMOs proving the need for a power which their own professional body (the Royal College of Psychiatrists) has recommended should be introduced.

Leaving that aside, it must be questioned whether a new power is needed, or whether a realization of the extent of the existing powers would not avoid the need for such a power. As the Report recognzes, it is quite clear that many people have misunderstood the circumstances in which sections 2 and 3 of the Mental Health Act 1983 may be used, despite the absolute clarity of the statutory language. The new Code of Practice may lead to a recognition of the availability of the existing powers. Thus avoiding the need for a dramatic or serious deterioration in condition prior to considering re-admission to Hospital. It is not only paragraph 2.6 of the new Code which highlights this point, but other paragraphs also make clear that a person's health or safety may, themselves, be sufficient for the conditions of the Act to be satisfied. Paragraph 2.9 provides:

'A patient may be admitted under Sections 2 and 3 solely in the interests of his own health even if there is no risk to his own or other people's safety. Those assessing the patient must consider:

- any evidence suggesting that the patient's mental health will deteriorate if he does not receive treatment;
- the reliability of such evidence which may include the known history of the individual's mental disorder;
- the views of the patient and of any relatives or close friends, especially those living with the patient, about the likely course of his illness and the possibility of its improving;
- the impact that any future deterioration or lack of improvement would have on relatives or close friends, especially those living with the patient, including an assessment of his ability and willingness to cope;
- whether there are other methods of coping with the expected deterioration or lack of improvement.'

It is not, therefore, necessary to show that the person's admission to hospital is appropriate for the protection of others'. Nor is there ever a requirement that the person be dangerous prior to admission (see paragraph 2.8). On the other hand, it is hospital admission that would be contemplated, rather than the person remaining in the community, and compulsory admission at that.

Further, there are close similarities between the new power and guardianship [60]. Guardianship enables the guardian to determine where patients reside, and the places to which they must go where certain activities are carried out; and ensures that access to them is provided, amongst others, to a doctor and social worker [61]. However, guardianship is rarely used [62]. The suggestion is that this is in part because the power to require the patient to participate in the various activities, including medical treatment, is not available. However, this must be set beside the perception at the time of the 1983 Act that the powers of the guardian had to be made specific rather than general and these powers were chosen because under the 1959 Act there was a perception that the reason guardianship was not then being used was because the powers, including authorizing medical treatment, were too extensive [63].

With such divergences of perception, one conclusion which might be drawn is that there is a reluctance to use community powers when they are available, but there is likely to be a demand for them when they are not available. Further, if guardianship is not used, why should a supervised discharge arrangement be any more popular?

The Review Team proposes that section 17 leave be extended for up to one year. Were a proposal to be introduced, it might, in itself, solve most problems. It would be reasonable to suggest that such an amendment should be introduced first before any new power. An assessment of its efficacy could then be made, along with the other recommendation made and already considered. Whether a new power was actually necessary could then be considered in the light of the success or failure of that amendment. Since any new power involves a significant development and a major infringement upon personal liberty, it is submitted that a slower move towards a new power is appropriate.

Some people are reluctant to use the formal procedures of the Act because of their stigmatizing effect. In the current context such reluctance is inappropriate [64]. Properly resourced community care facilities might avoid many if not most cases of such deterioration that some action is necessitated. This approach means that people are trusted in the community and relied upon to take their own decisions, by which they can make clear their capacity to be responsible and to take thought through decisions. Since the creation of a new compulsory power is a major infringement on personal liberty, the burden must be on its proponents to establish the necessity for it.

Does the proposal comply with appropriate criteria?

Secondly, does the particular proposal comply with sensible and appropriate criteria for caring for and treating people with mental health problems? Here it can be particularly controversial as to what criteria might be chosen, but an analysis of the current proposal against the criteria of the Law Commission in its current exercise concerned with decision-making is fruitful. The priorities of the Royal College and of the Law Commission may well be different. In reality this may, of course, not be the case. The Law Commission explicitly states its value base for making recommendations in the field of decision-making, whereas the Review Team identifies arguments for and against a power, in the light of such factors as the restrictions imposed by the European Convention on Human Rights. As indicated earlier, the Law Commission gives top priority to the principle 'that people should be enable and encourage to take for themselves those decisions which they are able to take'.

Whether this principle or the other two principles are satisfied is open to considerable doubt. It is suggested that the onus lies upon proponents of a new power to make clear that these are principles with which their proposal is consistent and that the extent to which there is interference with autonomy is predicated upon an objectively justifiable basis. Indeed, as Fennell [65] has pointed out, an earlier proposal by the Royal College of Psychiatrists for a similar Community Treatment Order was open to criticism on the basis that it failed adequately to address the balance of the need to respect people's welfare and to respect their wishes. Part of the problem is that knowledge about the efficacy of the current protections for people with mental disorder within the Mental Health Act is very limited. It is, therefore, not possible to be sure that the protection that is provided is adequate in safeguarding the patient's legitimate interests, whilst at the same time permitting treatment on a paternalistic basis.

The need for a detailed assessment

Thirdly, are there issues about this particular proposal upon which improvements need to be made? For present purposes a detailed examination of the proposal is not appropriate.

The potential effect upon community nurses

Fourthly, how might this proposal affect community nurses? It is after all usually nurses or social workers who will actually undertake the supervision and not the psychiatrist. It is the nurses and social workers who will be involved on a day-to-day basis. The delicate balance operated by hospital nurses between the roles that they have as treater/carer/therapist on the one hand and custodian on the other hand may simply not possible to maintain within the context of a supervised discharge arrangement. If for no other reason, this could be because there are fewer people with power with whom the patient would come into contact in the community than in hospital, therefore greater stress is placed upon the relationship between those few people and the patient. At least one real problem is avoided by the current proposals: there will be no compulsory treatment in the community. But if not, is there a need for a new power at all? The debate will no doubt continue.

8.6 Notes and references

1. See, generally, Hoggett, B.M., *Mental Health Law*, 3rd edn., London: Sweet & Maxwell, 1990; Gostin, L.O, *Mental Health Services: Law & Practice*, Looseleaf, Shaw & Sons: London; and Jones, R.M. *Mental Health Act Manual*, 4th edn., London: Sweet & Maxwell, 1994.
2. Mental Health Act Commission, *Fifth Biennial Report 1991–1993*, London: HMSO, 1993: para 7.15.
2a. See now *R* v. *South Western Hospital Managers, ex parte M.* [1994] 1 All ER 161.
3. See Fennell, P.W.H., 'Inscribing Paternalism in the Law: Consent to Treatment and Mental Disorder.' *Journal of Law & Society* 1990; 17; 29–51; pp 36–7 and Mental Health Act Commission, *Fifth Biennial Report 1991–1993*, London: HMSO, 1993: para 7.2.
4. Over the two year period 1 July 1991 to 30 June 1993, 46 patients were referred to the Mental Health Act Commission under section 57, which is significantly lower than in previous years: Mental Health Act Commission, *Fifth Biennial Report 1991–1993*, London: HMSO, 1993: para 7.2.

5. See Fennell, P.W.H., 'Inscribing Paternalism in the Law: Consent to Treatment and Mental Disorder.' *Journal of Law & Society* 1990; 17; 29–51; pp 37–40 and Mental Health Act Commission, *Fifth Biennial Report 1991–1993*, London: HMSO, 1993: paras 7.3 to 7.11 and 7.13 to 7.26.

6. This is indicated by the fact that, in the period 1991–1993, there were 4627 second opinion requests to the Mental Health Act Commission for medicines and 4067 for ECT, Mental Health Act Commission, *Fifth Biennial Report 1991–1993*, London: HMSO, 1993: Appendix 12, table 5.

7. The new edition of the Code of Practice came into force on 1 November 1993. The Mental Health Act does not impose a legal duty to comply with the Code 'but failure to follow the Code could be referred to in evidence in legal proceedings': Department of Health and Welsh Office, *Code of Practice: Mental Health Act 1983*, London: HMSO, 1993: para 1.1.

8. Where treatment is given under section 57 or under section 58 with a confirmatory second opinion (i.e. a Form 39 applies), there is a statutory scheme of review, see section 61, Code of Practice, paras 16.21 and 16.22 and Mental Health Act Commission, *Fifth Biennial Report 1991–1993*, London: HMSO, 1993: para 7.10. See also Mental Health Act Commission, *Fourth Biennial Report 1989–1991*, London: HMSO, 1991; para 6.4.

9. Section 59 of the Act and see Department of Health and Welsh Office, *Code of Practice: Mental Health Act 1983*, London: HMSO, 1993: para 16.15.

10. Department of Health and Welsh Office, *Code of Practice: Mental Health Act 1983*, London: HMSO, 1993: para 16.20.

11. See also Mental Health Act Commission, *Fifth Biennial Report 1991–1993*, London: HMSO, 1993: paras 7.7, 7.13 and 7.23.

12. Department of Health and Welsh Office, *Code of Practice: Mental Health Act 1983*, London: HMSO, 1993: paras 16.9 and 16.10 and Mental Health Act Commission, *Fifth Biennial Report 1991–1993*, London: HMSO, 1993: para 7.24.

13. Fennell, P.W.H., 'Inscribing Paternalism in the Law: Consent to Treatment and Mental Disorder.' *Journal of Law & Society* 1990; 17; 29–51; p 40 and Mental Health Act Commission, *Fifth Biennial Report 1991–1993*, London: HMSO, 1993: para 7.8.

14. Fennell, P.W.H., 'Inscribing Paternalism in the Law: Consent to Treatment and Mental Disorder.' *Journal of Law & Society* 1990; 17; 29–51; p 40.

15. Mental Health Act Commission, *Fifth Biennial Report 1991–1993*, London: HMSO, 1993: para 7.12.

16. Note the general concerns expressed in the Mental Health Act Commission, *Fifth Biennial Report 1991–1993*, London: HMSO, 1993: para 7.13.

17. Mental Health Act Commission, *Fourth Biennial Report 1989–1991*, London: HMSO, 1991; para 6.18. A Practice Note is now promised by the Commission, see Mental Health Act Commission, *Fifth Biennial Report 1991–1993*, London: HMSO, 1993: para 7.20.

18. Mental Health Act Commission, *Fifth Biennial Report 1991–1993*, London: HMSO, 1993: para 7.20.

19. *South West Hertfordshire H.A. v. Brady.* [1994] 2 *Med. Law Review* 208, recently confirmed by the Court of Appeal. See also *B. v. Croydon Health Authority* (1994) *The Times* December 1.

20. Department of Health and Welsh Office, *Code of Practice: Mental Health Act 1983*, London: HMSO, 1993.

21. As required by the decision in *F. v. West Berkshire Health Authority* (1989). See Practice Note (Sterilisation) [1993] 3 All ER 222.

22. A point made by Gillian Douglas in *Family Law* 1991; p 310.

23. Fennell, P.W.H., 'Inscribing Paternalism in the Law: Consent to Treatment and Mental Disorder.' *Journal of Law & Society 1990*; 17; 29–51; p 29.

24. Fennell, P.W.H., 'Inscribing Paternalism in the Law: Consent to Treatment and Mental Disorder.' *Journal of Law & Society 1990*; 17; 29–51; p 43.

25. The Law Commission, *Mentally Incapacitated Adults and Decision-Making: Medical Treatment and Research* (Consultation Paper No. 129), London: HMSO, 1993. For a critical appreciation of this document see Kennedy, I. and Grubb, A. 'The Law Commission's Proposals: An Introduction', [1994] 2 *Med. Law Review* 1; Gunn, M.' The Meaning of Incapacity', [1994] 2 *Med. Law Review* 8; Fennell, P. 'Statutory Authority to Treat Relatives and Treatment Proxies', [1994] 2 *Med. Law Review* 30; Stern, K. 'Advance Directives', [1994] 2 *Med. Law Review* 57; and Freeman, M. 'Deciding for the Intellectually Impaired', [1994] 2 *Med. Law Review* 77.

26. The Law Commission, *Mentally Incapacitated Adults and Decision-Making: Medical Treatment and Research* (Consultation Paper No. 129), London: HMSO, 1993: para 1.4.

27. The Law Commission, *Mentally Incapacitated Adults and Decision-Making: Medical Treatment and Research* (Consultation Paper No. 129), London: HMSO, 1993: para 1.5.

28. The Law Commission, *Mentally Incapacitated Adults and Decision-Making: Medical Treatment and Research* (Consultation Paper No. 129), London: HMSO, 1993: para 1.10.

29. The Law Commission, *Mentally Incapacitated Adults and Decision-Making: Medical Treatment and Research* (Consultation Paper No. 129), London: HMSO, 1993: paras 2.3 to 2.24.

30. The Law Commission, *Mentally Incapacitated Adults and Decision-Making: Medical Treatment and Research* (Consultation Paper No. 129), London: HMSO, 1993: para 3.40.

31. The Law Commission, *Mentally Incapacitated Adults and Decision-Making: Medical Treatment and Research* (Consultation Paper No. 129), London: HMSO, 1993: para 3.56.

32. The Law Commission, *Mentally Incapacitated Adults and Decision-Making: Medical Treatment and Research* (Consultation Paper No. 129), London: HMSO, 1993: paras 3.62 to 3.64.

33. The Law Commission, *Mentally Incapacitated Adults and Decision-Making: Medical Treatment and Research* (Consultation Paper No. 129), London: HMSO, 1993: para 4.4.

34. The Law Commission, *Mentally Incapacitated Adults and Decision-Making: Medical Treatment and Research* (Consultation Paper No. 129), London: HMSO, 1993: para 4.9.

35. The Law Commission, *Mentally Incapacitated Adults and Decision-Making: Medical Treatment and Research* (Consultation Paper No. 129), London: HMSO, 1993: para 4.10.

36. The Law Commission, *Mentally Incapacitated Adults and Decision-Making: Medical Treatment and Research* (Consultation Paper No. 129), London: HMSO, 1993: para 4.12.

37. The Law Commission, *Mentally Incapacitated Adults and Decision-Making: Medical Treatment and Research* (Consultation Paper No. 129), London: HMSO, 1993: para 4.13.

38. The Law Commission, *Mentally Incapacitated Adults and Decision-Making: Medical Treatment and Research* (Consultation Paper No. 129), London: HMSO, 1993: para 4.16.

39. The Law Commission, *Mentally Incapacitated Adults and Decision-Making: Medical Treatment and Research* (Consultation Paper No. 129), London: HMSO, 1993: para 4.20.

40. The Law Commission, *Mentally Incapacitated Adults and Decision-Making: Medical Treatment and Research* (Consultation Paper No. 129), London: HMSO, 1993: paras 4.28 and 4.29.

41. The Law Commission, *Mentally Incapacitated Adults and Decision-Making: Medical Treatment and Research* (Consultation Paper No. 129), London: HMSO, 1993: para 4.30.

42. The Law Commission, *Mentally Incapacitated Adults and Decision-Making: Medical Treatment and Research* (Consultation Paper No. 129), London: HMSO, 1993: para 6.23.

43. The Law Commission, *Mentally Incapacitated Adults and Decision-Making: Medical Treatment and Research* (Consultation Paper No. 129), London: HMSO, 1993: paras 6.3 to 6.14.

44. See Dimond, B., 'The Right of the Nurse to Detain Informal Patients in Psychiatric Hospitals in England and Wales.' *Medical Law* 1989; 8; p 535–47.

45. This means nurses who are registered in Part 3 (first level nurses trained in the nursing of persons suffering from mental illness) or Part 5 (first level nurses trained in the nursing of persons suffering from mental handicap) or Part 13 (nurses qualified following a course of preparation in mental health nursing) or Part 14 (nurses qualified following a course of preparation in mental handicap nursing): Mental Health (Nurses) Order 1983, S.I. 1983 No. 891, as amended in 1993 to included nurses trained under the UKCC Project 2000.

46. As it was described by David Lanham in an article of that title in *Criminal Law Review* 1974; p 515.

47. Confederation of Health Service Employees, *The Management of Violent or Potentially Violent Patients*, COHSE, 1977.

48. As to time out, see Department of Health and Welsh Office, *Code of Practice: Mental Health Act 1983* London: HMSO, 1993: chapter 19.

49. Department of Health and Welsh Office, *Code of Practice: Mental Health Act 1983* London: HMSO, 1993: para 18.15.

50. Ashworth Committee of Inquiry, *Report of the Committee of Inquiry*

into *Complaints about Ashworth Hospital* (Cm 2028–1), London: HMSO, 1993: p 205.

51. See also, Gunn, M.J., 'Judicial Review of Admission to Hospital and Treatment in the Community.' *Journal of Social Welfare Law* 1986; p 290.

52. Department of Health, *Legal Powers on the Care of Mentally Ill People in the Community*, London: Department of Health, 1993.

53. Royal College of Psychiatrists, *Community Supervision Orders*, London: Royal College of Psychiatrists, 1993.

54. Department of Health, *Legal Powers on the Care of Mentally Ill People in the Community*, London: Department of Health, 1993: para 2.7.

55. Department of Health, *Legal Powers on the Care of Mentally Ill People in the Community*, London: Department of Health, 1993: para 9.2.

56. Department of Health, *Legal Powers on the Care of Mentally Ill People in the Community*, London: Department of Health, 1993: para 7.14.

57. Department of Health, *Legal Powers on the Care of Mentally Ill People in the Community*, London: Department of Health, 1993: paras 8.7 and 8.8. This extension is to be found in the Mental Health Bill 1994.

58. Department of Health, *Legal Powers on the Care of Mentally Ill People in the Community*, London: Department of Health, 1993: para 8.8.

58a. The supervised discharge arrangement is to be introduced through the Mental Health Bill 1994.

59. Department of Health, *Legal Powers on the Care of Mentally Ill People in the Community*, London: Department of Health, 1993: para 8.14. Note that supervision registers have been introduced by circular, see HSG(95)5 and new guidance has been issued on the discharge of mentally disordered people, see HSG(94)27.

60. Sections 7 and 8 of the Mental Health Act 1983.

61. Section 8(2) of the Mental Health Act 1983.

62. Department of Health, *Legal Powers on the Care of Mentally Ill People in the Community*, London: Department of Health, 1993: para 7.13.

63. See Gunn, M.J., 'Mental Health Act Guardianship: Where Now?' *Journal of Social Welfare Law* 1986; pp 144–52.

64. Note the discussion of the importance of resources, see Department of Health, *Legal Powers on the Care of Mentally Ill People in the Community*, London: Department of Health, 1993: chapter 4.

65. Fennell, P.W.H., 'Inscribing Paternalism in the Law: Consent to Treatment and Mental Disorder.' *Journal of Law & Society* 1990; 17; 29–51; p 48–9.

B An Ethical Perspective – Compulsion in the Community
Harry Lesser

Professor Gunn's excellent survey of the five legal issues that he takes up raise many philosophical issues as well. I shall focus on one in particular: whether compulsory treatment and/or compulsory supervision within the community would be desirable. It will be convenient to consider these separately, and in the case of compulsory treatment to consider separately issues of principle and practicability.

8.7 Compulsory treatment

8.7.1 *Issues of principle*

The most thoroughgoing of objections in principle, which would apply equally to compulsory treatment in institutions, is the objection of Thomas Szasz [1] and others that there is no such thing as mental illness. By this, Szasz means that all those who injure themselves or others, however bizarre the circumstances, nevertheless act out of a free choice, and not because their mental judgement is impaired. Hence, though they may legitimately be punished for harming other people, like other criminals, they may not be restrained in advance, on the ground that they might be a danger to themselves or others, any more than any other person who has committed no crime.

Szasz's objections

The basic assumption here is that no one is so mentally impaired as to lose responsibility for their actions (or virtually no one – Szasz does admit that a very few people are so incapable of making decisions that one has to act on their behalf, as one must when a patient is unconscious). It is not clear that this can be absolutely disproved; but one can say that the empirical evidence, both from the behaviour of 'mentally disturbed' people and from subsequent reports by those who have been 'mentally ill', *is* strongly against it. Nevertheless, though few people agree with Szasz, he has called attention to two important points

- that it is not always easy to decide when someone is so mentally disturbed and potentially dangerous as to require compulsory treatment, and
- that in the past many people have been unnecessarily committed to mental institutions.

Although I think Szasz's objection should be rejected, on empirical grounds if for no other reason, these points should still be kept in mind in any discussion of the rights and wrongs of compulsory treatment.

Control through drugs

However, this leads to another objection, this time specifically against compulsory treatment in the community. It might be argued that, once we accept that compulsory treatment can be legitimate, then either a person is so disturbed as to need it or they are not. If they do need it, they also need, hopefully only temporarily, to be confined to an institution, for the protection of themselves and others; if they are not so disturbed as to need committal to a mental hospital, they are by the same token not sufficiently disturbed to justify being treated compulsorily. One cannot, it might be said, have things both ways.

What this ignores, though, is the ability that now exists to control mental illness through drugs. To what extent mental illness is amenable to this treatment is a very controversial matter; but again there is strong empirical evidence that some conditions in some patients can be cured in this way, and some can be controlled, though not cured. This means that these are people who can cope with life in the community, and are not dangerous to themselves or others, but only as long as they take their medication. For such people, compulsory treatment in the community would be in principle justifiable, though it might still turn out to be undesirable or impracticable.

Yet this may be too simple, as Professor Gunn's own objection to it suggests. Professor Gunn says (section 8.5.4): 'Since the creation of a new compulsory power is a major infringement on personal liberty, the burden must be on its proponents to establish the necessity for it'.

Infringement on liberty or not?

This raises several points. First, though one should agree that it is for the proponents to establish that the power is needed, it is not clear that to introduce this power would be a major infringement of liberty, since a more severe power, that of compulsory detention in an institution, already exists. To this one might reply that this assumes that the power would be used only over people who would otherwise be in institutions, whereas it might well be used over people who would be living in the community subject to no special restrictions at all: it *could* be used actually to limit the infringement of liberty, but could also do the reverse. It could still be reasonably maintained that the restriction on liberty that is involved is not very great; but it would seem to be great enough for the onus of proof to be on those who wish to introduce it.

Given this, has the case been made? Professor Gunn gives two reasons why it has not, which are hinted at in the above quote, but made more explicit elsewhere in his chapter. First, though he would agree, (I think) that cases of the kind described above do occur, there is some uncertainty about their frequency. Apart from 'anecdotal evidence ... and the evidence of a number of highly publicized incidents' (section 8.5.4) there is what might cynically be regarded as one professionally biased survey. We do not know that there really is a substantial problem which requires a new form of action. Secondly, he holds that it has not been shown that existing powers, properly used, are insufficient.

Consequences of ignoring the problem

On the first point, given the harm done in these cases, which includes murder, permanent physical damage, and the creation of unbearable levels of fear and stress for relatives and neighbours even when the mentally disturbed person is threatening and unpredictable rather than violent, there is a need to tackle them even if they are relatively few in number. It is worth noting that the fact that a case is put emotively does not invalidate it, unless (for example) what is not harmful is being described as if it were: here, where the harm is genuine, to refer to it in emotive terms may be unnecessary but does not alter the facts. Nor is it necessarily inappropriate to be anecdotal: it is inappropriate if one is seeking to establish that something is a general rule or is widespread, but appropriate if, as here, one is merely trying to show that it does sometimes happen and measures should be taken to deal with it – for which purpose a scientific case in unnecessary.

But Professor Gunn's second point is valid. If what I have argued so far is correct, there is a real problem concerning people who are mentally disturbed, likely to injure themselves or others and yet not in institutions – some of them, moreover, need not be in institutions if it can be guaranteed that they take their medication regularly. The problem may not involve many people, but it exists; and the consequences of ignoring it are terrible. Compulsory treatment in the community has been proposed as one way of dealing with it: and I have argued that it is justifiable in principle. But we still have to ask

(1) whether it is necessary, or whether, as Professor Gunn argues, existing powers are sufficient to deal with the problem, and
(2) whether it is in any case practicable.

8.7.2 Issues of practicality

Possibilities

That it is in the strict sense practicable is shown by the fact that it is in operation in two places – the state of Victoria in Australia and Madison, Wisconsin in the USA. Not much is yet known about its success, but in Madison it forms part of the programme of care in the community into which considerable resources have been put, and the feeling seems to be that it could not work without such resources. This emphasizes Professor Gunn's point about its necessity. For one could suggest that if

(1) we were more ready to commit people to institutions when necessary and
(2) proper resources were provided for community care, as at the moment they certainly are not,

then by one means or the other the problem would be dealt with – either by 'greater preparedness to use the Mental Health Act earlier than is often the case', or by 'properly resourced community care facilities.' (section 8.5.4).

It would certainly seem that if community 'care' really were care, and if resources were provided to make this possible, then many of those people who should not be in institutions but do need help and treatment would be able to cope with their own lives, behave in ways that are tolerable, and keep up their medication. Since the Madison experience suggests that compulsory treatment, if used at all, cannot be a substitute for well-resourced community care (as the government may be hoping), but on the contrary depends on its availability if it is to work, the first priority should be to work to improve resources for community care. This is in no way incompatible with also having compulsory treatment if it is still needed. But in the present political climate, probably it is a matter of one or the other. It follows, therefore, that at the moment, when compulsory treatment may well be seized on as an excuse for not improving resources, it should probably be opposed, and concentration should rather be on trying to get proper resources.

But this needs to be qualified. First, if it ever becomes certain or near-certain that the resources will not be forthcoming, compulsory treatment might well be the least bad option, particularly if there is also a continuing refusal to be more ready to put people in institutions. Secondly, there may still be a small number of people who do not need to be in institutions but even with good community care either cannot or will not respond properly on their own account: in other words, though I agree with Professor Gunn that existing procedures and better resources would greatly reduce the problem, I am not convinced that they would eliminate it. There could still be people potentially dangerous to themselves or others who simply cannot be persuaded to take their medication voluntarily, even though there might not be many of them. Hence, even though improving resources should be the first priority, because it is likely to do the most good and relieve the most harm, compulsory treatment may still be desirable at least as a last resort and for a few people.

Problems

Even here, though, Professor Gunn has made three important objections. Explicitly, he points out that, though a hospital mental nurse may be able to act both as a carer and as a custodian, in the community the double role may be impossible to maintain. We must ask whether it is right to require community nurses to inject people in their own homes. Implicitly, he suggests, I think, both that compulsory treatment would interfere with the attempt to 'rehabilitate' people precisely by genuinely trusting them and that the power, once granted, might be used more widely than it should.

All these are indeed possible dangers. The first, though, can be partly dealt with by having community supervision of a compulsory kind, but no compulsory treatment in the community. Those who refused to comply with the supervision order would be returned to the institution rather than compulsorily injected in their own homes.

8.8 Compulsory supervision

This is in fact what has been advocated by the Royal College of Psychiatrists in their proposal [2]. I indicated at the beginning of this comment that it would be convenient to consider compulsory treatment and compulsory supervision separately, although up to now I have discussed compulsory treatment. One may now suggest that there may well be good reasons for rejecting compulsory treatment in the community, as the College do, while accepting the case for compulsory supervision. This not only reduces the custodial role of the nurse to a workable level, but also interferes less with the freedom of the 'patient', and allows them to retain as much autonomy as may help them to establish themselves back in the community, and perhaps as much as they can cope with. Finally, the details of the proposal go a long way towards ensuring that the orders would only be used when appropriate.

8.9 Conclusions

My tentative conclusions are therefore as follows. There is no objection in principle to compulsory treatment in the community for those who are mentally disturbed and a potential danger to themselves or others, provided that they are correctly identified. There is however a strong objection in practice, because this might well interfere with the relationship between nurse and patient in a way very detrimental to good nursing. Moreover, compulsory supervision would serve the same purpose, while being less objectionable. Hence, there is a strong case for introducing compulsory supervision orders, e.g. on the lines suggested by the College.

8.9.1 *The need for resources*

However, this is appropriate only in a very small number of cases. For I agree with Professor Gunn that most of the problems for which compulsory treatment and supervision are proposed as solutions would be better dealt with by more use of existing powers and by much better community resources. Accordingly, I have suggested that our first priority should be to seek better resources: if this fails, or if there is still a problem even if it succeeds, community supervision could be the next step.

8.9.2 *Autonomy or welfare*

Finally, we need to consider a more theoretical point, though it may have practical consequences. Should consideration of these questions be governed by the principles laid down in the Law Commission's document on *Mentally Incapacitated Adults and Decision-Making* [3] or those laid down by the Reed Committee and accepted by the Royal College of Psychiatrists [4]? The Law Commission give top priority to autonomy (though the word is not used) and to the ability to take one's own decisions, and hold that intervention should be limited to what is absolutely necessary. The Reed Committee make the patient's welfare, the quality of care and attention to their individual needs, the top priority, though they are concerned to maximize independence and minimize institutional control, as part of this. These could lead to very much the same result in practice, since both sets of principles hold, in effect, that wherever people are capable of making decisions for themselves they should be allowed and encouraged to do so. Nevertheless, there is a difference of emphasis. Indeed, Professor Gunn argues (section 8.5.4) that the proposals of the College are incompatible with the principles laid down by the Law Commission. It is not clear that they are: compulsory supervision orders could be seen as an excellent example of the kind of necessary, minimal intervention prescribed in their second principle [5]. But the fact that he argues in this way shows that it may be quite important to consider whether autonomy or welfare should be the ultimate value.

In considering this question, we have to bear in mind the terrible interference with the autonomy of mental patients that has gone on in the past, and still exists, both in the committal to institutions of people who either were not ill or could cope better in their own homes and in the gross under-estimation of what *some* mentally ill people can still do. But we must not fall into the opposite error, of treating people as autonomous when in fact they cannot take proper decisions: to do so is just as cruel and stupid as to deny autonomy to those who can use it. Moreover, the danger at the moment is precisely here: whereas once people were in institutions who should not have been, now people remain in the community who need to be in hospital. There is therefore a practical reason, at the moment, for regarding the Reed Committee's principles as better judged.

There is also, perhaps more importantly, a basic theoretical reason. It is not clear that autonomy is in itself of value: it is valuable because adults are normally the best judges of their own interests (imperfect judges, but better than other people who are not in their situation), because we simply cannot be trusted with power over each other, and because taking control of one's life makes one (often though not always) more satisfied, stronger minded, more intelligent and of more use to oneself and others. But this last point is to say that autonomy is a means, not an end; and therefore that, though people must be allowed to take risks and to do what other people consider foolish, to limit a person's autonomy in the name of their welfare may not be always unjust – though it always sets a dangerous example. If this is so, in principle, even perhaps for the mentally well, it is clearly so once a person's judgment is so impaired that they are not in fact taking autonomous decisions. It is therefore right that welfare should be the supreme goal (and not only the welfare of the individual patient, but also of those they may injure), and that autonomy should be respected only when it genuinely exists, and can contribute to a person's welfare. We should be cautious about limiting autonomy in the name of welfare, but be quite clear that it is sometimes the right thing to do.

Accordingly, I would suggest in conclusion, and in contrast to Professor Gunn, that the proposals from the Royal College of Psychiatrists are in principle sound. But I would agree with Professor Gunn that they could be legitimately applied only to a small number of people, perhaps a very small number; and I would also agree that the first things to be done are to increase the use of existing legal powers and to improve the resources for community care, after which comparatively little of the problem, one hopes, would remain.

8.10 Notes and references

Acknowledgement

I am very grateful to Ms. Caroline Dunn, Ph.D. student at Manchester University, for information about the situation in Madison.

1. Szasz, T., *The myth of mental illness*. London: Secker & Warburg, 1962.
2. Royal College of Psychiatrists, *Community Supervision Orders*. London: Royal College of Psychiatrists, 1993.
3. The Law Commission, *Mentally Incapacitated Adults and Decision-*

Making: Medical Treatment and Research (Consultation Paper No. 129). London: HMSO, 1993.

4. Royal College of Psychiatrists, *Community Supervision Orders*. London: Royal College of Psychiatrists, 1993.

5. The Law Commission, *Mentally Incapacitated Adults and Decision-Making: Medical Treatment and Research* (Consultation Paper No. 129). London: HMSO, 1993, at para. 1.4.

Chapter 9
The Critically Ill Patient

A The Legal Perspective
Diana Brahams

9.1 General principles

9.1.1 *Court involvement in medical treatment in general*

Increasingly, in the last decade, the Courts have been invited to offer guidance in relation to medical treatment and decision making or to consider and judge the conduct of the doctors and other medical staff having responsibility for the care of patients and also at times to challenge the level of treatment resources on offer to an individual patient or class of patient (though these are not usually successful) [1]. By contrast, the Courts have also been invited to approve discontinuance of treatment so as to allow a patient to die where the prognosis is hopeless and continued active treatment is thought to provide no benefit at all (*Airedale NHS Trust v. Bland* (1993).

The age of the patients concerned ranges from attempts to protect unborn babies (whose mothers' behaviour or unwillingness to have treatment looks to put the baby's health and safety before, during and after birth at risk (see section 9.4.3) [2] new born babies and children under the age of 18 (who are subject to the wardship jurisdiction of the High Court and also the Children Act 1989) to decisions for the old and senile. The range is across the entire spectrum of patients, from young, adult and either lucid or mentally incapable to the old, feeble, infirm and moribund. The law regulates and even limits many aspects of medical practice and conduct (in England and Wales it remains a crime to aid, abet, counsel or procure a suicide notwithstanding that suicide itself is no longer a crime). Other examples of where the law regulates medical practice can be found in particular, in the areas of reproductive medicine, e.g. abortion, surrogacy and the procedures governed by the Human Fertilisation and Embryology Act 1990.

9.1.2 *Sources of the legal principles*

The fundamental principles of English common law (and much of statute) stem from Judaeo-Christian concepts of morality as propounded, developed and applied by judges over the centuries. In addition there is the impact of EC law and directives on domestic law and practice.

Enshrined in UK law and practice (subject to a number of exceptions) is the principle of sanctity of life and the duty, where possible and appropriate, to preserve life, but this must be considered alongside the autonomy of the individual and the right of a capable lucid individual to decide what shall be done to his own body (subject to overriding by the state, e.g. in war or to protect the community at large, and subject to resource availability and prioritizing of treatments).

9.1.3 Consent

Where a patient is mentally capable his permission must be sought and obtained appropriately before treatment can lawfully be provided. If there is an emergency and a patient is unconscious, then, subject to no contra-indications being found or known to the doctors, treatment may be given to preserve life and health.

Minors

The Family Law Reform Act 1969, section 8 provides that children aged 16 and over can consent to medical and dental treatment as if of full age (but not necessarily refuse it) and the common law allows for consent (and where appropriate refusal of treatment) where a child is sufficiently intellectually mature and intelligent to understand and have insight into the treatment on offer (*Gillick* v. *West Norfolk and Wisbech Area Health Authority* (1985). Parents of a child under 18 can give consent as can the Court in Wardship and see also the Children Act 1989. The consent for or refusal of treatment must be made independently and freely and not under duress or the undue influence of another person (such as a parent or relative as in *Re T* (1992).).

Fluctuating capacity

Where a person's ability to understand may vary over time, the answer to a question whether or not the patient has the capacity to consent or refuse treatment may depend upon the time at which that question is asked. Where the person's understanding fluctuates or may improve in the future, and the treatment can safely be delayed, it is appropriate for the medical staff to seek the patient's views and to assess capacity when his understanding is at its best. (See also section 6.2.2.)

Mental incapacity

Where a patient aged over 18 is so mentally incapacitated that he or she cannot give a valid consent or refusal to treatment, the doctors and medical staff caring for that patient must act reasonably in accordance with what they reasonably understand to be in that patient's best interests. (See also sections 8.2.1 and 8.2.2.) The question of whether the medical staff have acted reasonably is judged by the test laid down in *Bolam* v. *Friern Hospital Management Committee* (1957) the standard applied is to assess whether or not a doctor or other professional person's conduct was in accordance with a practice thought proper by a responsible body of medical opinion [3].

9.2 Mental incapacity

9.2.1 Special category treatments

Where the treatment falls within a special category (e.g. sterilization, organ donation, medical research, etc.) it is appropriate for the medical carers to seek approval in the form of a declaration of legality from the High Court, though a failure to do so will not of itself render appropriate treatment unlawful (*F* v. *West Berkshire Health Authority* (1990)). However, in such cases where the patient is aged less than 18 it is mandatory to obtain the approval of the High Court in Wardship or otherwise (*Re B* (1987)).

9.2.2 Intervention in adult cases limited to Mental Health Act powers

Originally the courts had an inherent *parens patriae* jurisdiction similar to that now exercised in wardship which extended to all incapacitated persons but which was revoked, probably by mistake, by the Mental Health Act 1959. The common law now provides no grounds on which the court or any other person can validly consent to treatment for anything other than a mental disorder for mentally incapacitated adults under the Mental Health Act 1983 (see section 8.1), though the courts have an inherent jurisdiction to declare treatments as lawful if they consider it appropriate. There is an excellent up-to-date review of the law relating to medical decision making in respect of the mentally incapacitated adult in the Law Commission's Consultation Paper *Mentally Incapacitated Adults and Decision-Making* [4].

9.2.3 Where the courts decline jurisdiction

There may be other decisions relating to medical treatment which fall outside the 'special' category but for which some independent confirmation is appropriate. In the case of in *Re GF* (1992), Sir Stephen

Brown, President of the Family Division, held that the court did not have to intervene and grant a declaration where the effect of the operation, here a hysterectomy, was essentially therapeutic, despite the fact that the operation would result in the sterilization of the patient, provided that two medical practitioners were satisfied that the operation was necessary for therapeutic purposes, that it was in the best interests of the patient, and that there was no practicable less intrusive means of treating the condition. A similar approach might be developed for a range of treatments. In *Re: SG* (1991), Sir Stephen Brown said that there was no declaration required from the court to authorize an abortion on a mentally handicapped woman, as the law on abortion was already adequately covered by statute and, in particular, by the Abortion Act 1967 (as amended) a second opinion is required for an abortion to be carried out under the Act. (But see section 8.2.3.)

Similarly, in the case of in *Re: H* (1993), the court refused to grant a declaration effectively approving invasive medical treatment to be given to a 25-year old voluntary mental patient who was diagnosed as a chronic schizophrenic and who was an in-patient.

At the hearing the Official Solicitor agreed the procedures were lawful but opposed the summons on the basis that it was inappropriate for a court to make a declaration. It was held by the deputy judge sitting in the Family Division that the proposed invasive medical procedures were in the patient's best interests and were accordingly lawful, notwithstanding the patient's incapacity to consent to them. However, it was not essential to the lawfulness of the proposed operation for it to have been the subject of any declaration under the court's inherent jurisdiction. The court would not weigh up the risks of vexatious litigation by a patient who recovered from mental illness in deciding whether to exercise the discretion to grant a declaration.

The proper principle to apply in deciding whether to grant a declaration was in the interests of all other doctors and all other mental patients in relation to whom an analogous situation might arise in the future. A declaration by the Court that the procedures proposed were lawful might be an unfortunate signal to others in the future that it was appropriate as a matter of good medical practice for the implementation of such procedures to be delayed pending the outcome of a costly application to the court. This decision makes it clear that unnecessary application for treatments which fall outside the defined serious categories or which are not otherwise distinctly controversial should not form the basis of applications to the court which does not wish to participate in or take responsibility for day-to-day decision-making which is best left to the medical carers and the patient's family after considering what is in the individual patient's best interests. These are cases which fall outside the very serious cases where the court's approval is appropriate, such as *Airedale NHS Trust* v. *Bland* (1993).

9.2.4 The Law Commission guidelines

As to that, guidance is to be found in the Law Commission's Consultation Paper 129 [5] in its proposals as to a best interest criteria whereby:

'consideration should be given to:

(1) the ascertainable past and present wishes and feelings (considered the light of his or her understanding at the time) of the incapacitated person;

(2) whether there is an alternative to the proposed treatment, and in particular whether there is an alternative which is more conservative or which is less intrusive or restrictive;

(3) the factors which the incapacitated person might be expected to consider if able to do so, including the likely effect of the treatment on the person's life expectancy, health, happiness, freedom and dignity . . .

The interests of people other than the incapacitated person should not be considered except to the extent that they have a bearing on the incapacitated person's individual interests.'

9.2.5 Omission not commission

In *Airedale NHS Trust* v. *Bland* (1993) the withdrawal of medical treatment (in this case artificial hydration and nutrition) was held to take the form of a legal omission rather than commission.

The successive courts who heard the arguments in *Airedale NHS Trust* v. *Bland* were at pains to make it clear that the issues under discussion and review bore no relation to euthanasia and contrasted the case of *R* v. *Cox* (1993) where a consultant physician was found guilty of the attempted murder of a dying patient to whom he had administered a potassium chloride injection. The patient was in unbearable pain but the Court held that the doctor's intention had not been to relieve pain and in so doing shorten her life but to end life. Had Dr Cox used a different means such as insulin or morphine which had pain killing qualities yet at the same time had shortened life even to the point of causing death within a short time of administration, his actions would have been lawful [6].

9.3 The Select Committee on Medical Ethics Report 1994

In *Airedale* v. *Bland*, a number of judges made it clear that they wished Parliament to review the situation with regard to treatment of hopelessly ill patients who may or may not be suffering great pain and in consequence of this case and also perhaps following on from the decision in *R* v. *Cox* (1993) a Select Committee of the House of Lords on medical ethics was appointed to consider [7]

> 'The ethical, legal and clinical implications of the person's right to withhold consent to life-prolonging treatment, and the position of persons who are no longer able to give or withhold consent; and to consider whether and in what circumstances actions that have as their intention or a likely consequence the shortening of another person's life may be justified on the grounds that they accord with that person's wishes or with that person's best interests; and in all the foregoing considerations to pay regard to the likely effects of changes in law or medical practice on society as a whole.'

9.3.1 *The supremacy of the patient's views*

The report, published in 1994, [8]

> 'strongly endorsed the right of the competent patient to refuse consent to any medical treatment, for whatever reason. The doctor must ensure that the patient understands the likely consequence of such refusal, and the reasons for proposing a particular treatment, but no member of the health-care team may overrule the patient's decision ... we urge that, if an individual refusal of treatment is overruled by the Court, full reasons should be given.'

9.3.2 *Euthanasia*

The Committee felt that there was insufficient reason to weaken society's prohibition of intentional killing and recommended against a change in the law so as to permit euthanasia as it would

> 'not be possible to set secure limits on voluntary euthanasia and to create an exception to the general rule against intentional killing would be to open the door to its further erosion.... The law should not distinguish between 'murder and mercy killing' as it would cross the line which prohibits any intentional killing, a line which we think it is essential to preserve.'

The most recent developments in Holland which are widening the categories of permissible euthanasia in practice suggest these anxieties are well founded [9].

However, the Committee welcomed moves to ensure that senior doctors supervised casualty departments to discourage inappropriately aggressive treatment by the less experienced practitioners and at the same time strongly recommended the development and growth of palliative care services.

9.3.3 When to stop treatment

The Committee saw little ethical difference between stopping a treatment and not starting it and did not distinguish between withholding and withdrawal of treatment when considering decisions involving the limitation of treatment. There is a point at which the duty to try to save the patient's life is exhausted and at which continued treatment may be inappropriate. The problem is that there may be no consensus on when this point has been reached.

Where the patient was incompetent, 'treatment-limiting' decisions should be taken by all those involved in his or her care, including the entire health care team and the family or other people closest to the patient. Their guiding principle should be that a treatment may be judged inappropriate if it adds nothing to the patient's well-being as a person. It was not helpful to distinguish firmly between treatment and personal care which were both part of a continuum and such boundaries as exist between them shift as practice evolves and 'particularly as the wider role of nursing develops'.

The Committee was divided as to whether nutrition and hydration, even when given by invasive methods (as was in point in the Bland case) may ever be regarded as a treatment which in certain circumstances is inappropriate but was unanimous in agreeing that this question need not usually be asked.

> 'Progressive development and ultimate acceptance of the notion that some treatment is inappropriate should make it unnecessary to consider the withdrawal of nutrition and hydration, except in circumstances where its administration is evidently burdensome to the patient.'

9.3.4 Persistent vegetative state (PVS)

Frenchay Healthcare NHS Trust v. S

On January 14, 1994 the issue of withdrawal of feeding or failure to reinstate invasive feeding in a PVS patient was considered by the Court of Appeal in the case of *Frenchay Healthcare NHS Trust* v. *S* (1994). In that case the patient had been a healthy young man who, in June 1991, took a drug overdose which resulted in acute and irreversible brain damage diagnosed as PVS. Until June 1993 he was fed through a nasogastric tube but subsequently a gastrostomy tube was inserted through the stomach wall. On January 10, 1994 the tube had become disconnected. There was disagreement as to whether no further action should be taken and death allowed to supervene naturally or whether a further operation be undertaken to insert a new tube.

The question for the Court of Appeal was what was in the best interests of this patient. There was no reason to question the conclusion of his consultant that it was in his best interests for no further action to be taken and for him to die naturally. The appeal by the offical solicitor was dismissed.

The court suggested that where a hospital sought to discontinue the treatment of a PVS patient it should apply for and obtain a declaration that it was proper to do so. This has been formalized into a Practice Note. The procedures are similar to those relating to applications for sterilization for incompetent patients and expressly state that the High Court may determine the effect of a purported advance directive as to future medical treatment. 'In summary, the patient's previously expressed views, if any, will always be a very important component in the decisions of the doctors and the court.'

The patient's state of mind

The state of mind of S when he took a drug overdose did not emerge in the judgment in the *Frenchay* case. It is unclear whether the overdose was intentional or accidental and this was not put in issue. Arguably it could have been relevant when considering the views of the patient.

Accordingly, where a patient develops PVS due to a failed suicide attempt (but there was no evidence that he was mentally so disturbed or unbalanced that he could be judged to have been incompetent at the time of the act, whether temporarily or otherwise) then is there a deemed consent or refusal to firstly resuscitation and/or secondly maintenance in a PVS state? If the patient did not wish to live before he had PVS why should he be deemed willing to be maintained in such a state?

A definition

The Committee suggested the development of a generally accepted definition of what is PVS with a view to leading to a code of practice for patients in this state. Suggested elements to be included were:

'that over a period of not less than 12 months there had been no return of cognitive behavioural or verbal responses, no purposive motor responses or other evidence of voluntary motor activity ...'

Diagnosis should be on repeated observations of those criteria by the physician responsible for the care of the patient and confirmed by a neurologist of consultant status who had not been previously involved with the case.

9.3.5 *Advance directives*

The Committee also welcomed the development of advance directives but concluded that legislation was unnecessary as doctors increasingly recognised their ethical obligations to comply with them. Instead, a code of practice agreed between all the health care professions should be developed. The development of case law was moving in the same direction. The British Medical Association's Statement on advance directives would be a good basis for such a code [10].

The advance directive should be respected unless there were reasonable grounds to believe that the clinical circumstances prevailing were significantly different from those anticipated by the patient, or that the patient had changed his views since the directive was prepared. A directive could be overruled if it requests treatment not clinically indicated or any illegal action. Patients should be encouraged to review their directives regularly.

The Committee did not favour proxy decision making for incompetent patients and felt that decisions about the treatments which society can afford should be made away from the hospital ward or consulting room and on the basis that treatment should be available to all on an equal basis.

Similarly, in their Consultation Paper 129, the Law Commission were generally encouraging of the anticipatory decision making documents and under the heading 'The protection of treatment providers' [11] it stated that:

'Under the current law, we consider it unlikely that liability would be incurred for acts reasonably performed in accordance with a patient's valid anticipatory decision. Legitimate doubt may remain, however, in relation to cases where an anticipatory decision is subsequently shown to have been invalid. An example would be where it is later shown that the decision had already been revoked before it was acted on.'

Their proposal is that treatment providers who act in accordance with an apparently valid and continuing anticipatory decision would only be liable to any civil or criminal proceedings if they did so in bad faith or without resonable care.

9.4 Case study A – mother and/or baby

Let us now consider the application of these general principles in the context of two case scenarios.

Case A involves a woman in childbirth who is under the care of the midwife, a critically ill mother who refuses further treatment, including a caesarean and blood transfusion thought to be necessary to preserve her life of and that of the unborn child.

9.4.1 *The facts*

Mrs A was a practising Jehovah's Witness who did not believe in blood transfusions and liked to keep medical interventions to the minimum. Her husband felt similarly and this was know to their GP. Mrs A had arranged for a home confinement. There appeared to be no problems during pregnancy. When labour pains began Mrs A telephoned for the midwife who came some 40 minutes later. The pregnancy was at full term. Shortly after the midwife arrived the membranes ruptured spontaneously. Further examination indicated that the birth of the child was obstructed and that there were signs that the fetus was becoming distressed.

The midwife considered that Mrs. A should be taken to hospital as it seemed to her that a caesarean might be indicated and that without the provision of specialist care and facilities the mother's life and that of the baby would be at risk. She informed Mr. and Mrs. A that it was her intention to call for an ambulance and that it might be necessary to perform a caesarean though she was not in a position to say definitely one way or the other. The mother made it clear that she would not be willing to undergo a caesarean section and would die with her baby in childbirth if this was to be the alternative. The midwife asked if she would be willing to travel to hospital in an ambulance which was refused. The midwife then telephoned the GP and the obstetric and gynaecological department of the local hospital recounting the symptoms and her provisional diagnosis over the telephone and requesting support and advice. She decided to call an ambulance in any event.

When the ambulance came Mrs. A refused to travel in it at which point the GP appeared. He was unable to persuade Mrs. A to go in the ambulance to hospital. He summoned a specialist obstetrician to come out from the local hospital but this was some way away and it was not expected that the consultant would arrive for another hour at least by which time it was likely that irreversible brain damage would have occurred. The mother's condition was patently deteriorating and becoming critical as well.

9.4.2 *Legal issues raised and steps to be taken*

The duty of care

It is clear that the providers of health care owe Mrs. A and her unborn child a duty of care. Unfortunately, Mrs. A has made it clear that she has no intention of accepting the treatment which the midwife and the GP think would be in her and the baby's best interests. This does not mean that their duty of care towards her has come to an end and they are entitled to refuse to give her any treatment if she does not accept what they would wish her to have.

The need to inform

However, it is incumbent upon them to make the consequences of her refusal very clear and to do their best to persuade her (and in this case her husband who is likely to have influence) to go in the ambulance to hospital and submit to whatever invasive treatment including a caesarean section and if necessary a blood transfusion if this is deemed necessary. The problem for the GP and the midwife is that Mrs. A is so unco-operative that she will not even voluntarily go in the ambulance and they are faced with having to do the best they can with inadequate facilities and a lack of specialist help.

The need to keep records

It is important in such cases for the health carers to write full and coherent notes and to record the fact that they tried to persuade the patient to undergo appropriate treatment and that this was refused and the ground of a refusal if provided should be stated (here religious conviction).

Battery and false imprisonment

Should Mrs A's objections be overridden and she be forced into the ambulance against her will? If she were to resist being taken in the ambulance then such transportation would amount to false imprisonment and the manhandling necessary would amount to a trespass to the person and battery which could give rise to both a civil and criminal action. As already indicated, the law recognises the autonomy of the lucid adult patient and treatment which is not consensual becomes a battery.

Options to follow

The midwife and the GP left in charge of this difficult patient who has put both her life and that of her unborn child at risk must do the best that they can within their experience and the facilities available to them while at the same time seeking urgently more specialist help if such is available to ensure that all that can be done within the confines of the patient's refusal is done. Thus if it is possible (albeit risky) for an attempt to be made to deliver the baby vaginally with forceps or by some other means and this is the only manner of delivery permitted by the mother then this must be attempted and reasonable skill applied. At all times, as explained above, the medical health carers and in particular the midwife and the GP left with the patient until any specialist help can arrive must make the consequences of a refusal to undergo appropriate treatment very clear and record this.

Overriding duty to the child once born

If the baby is born alive, notwithstanding the difficulties, then any refusal by the mother to allow the baby to be taken to a specialist unit should be overridden in the interests of the child and subsequent application made in Wardship or as necessary to the High Court under the Children Act 1989.

9.4.3   *The basic dilemmas – (1) mother's convictions or the rights of the fetus?*

Are there any other options open to the midwife and the GP or any other medical health carer who comes on the scene? Does the fact that there is an unborn child whose life is endangered by the actions of its mother alter the situation? Should an application be made to the Family Division of the High Court? What would the likely result be?

English law

Strictly speaking under English law an unborn child has no individual legal status and cannot be heard or represented independently from its mother. In *Re F (in utero)* (1988) the Court of Appeal refused an application to make the fetus (almost at term) a ward of court so that it could be protected from its mother who had a past history of being unable to care adequately for a child, who led a nomadic existence and who, shortly before the child was due, again went missing. The application was refused both at first instance and in the Court of Appeal on the grounds that, until the child was actually born, there would be an inherent incompatibility between any projected exercise of the wardship jurisdiction and the rights and welfare of the mother. Relying on *Paton v. British Pregnancy Advisory Service Trustee* (1988), the Court of Appeal first concluded that the fetus had no individual personality and that, therefore, there could be no jurisdiction in wardship; secondly, it made it clear that in practice it would be impossible to follow the principle of the paramountcy in wardship of the child's welfare if that conflicted with the liberty and legal interest of the mother.

The American experience

Attempts to intervene against the wishes of the mother in the United States in the case of *AC* in 1987 illustrated very well the dangers of interventionism in this field. In that case, an American Court decided to force an unwanted caesarean on a 27-year old woman dying from cancer who was 26 weeks pregnant. She, her husband and her parents were wholly opposed to the operation and her usual doctor refused to perform it. Notwithstanding this, the Court made an order and another doctor was found to carry out the caesarean section. The baby died within hours and the mother died two days later in the bitter knowledge that her child had died and her dying wishes had been disregarded. The parents appealed, arguing that the operation had violated their daughter's bodily integrity, and they were supported by women's and religious groups, the American Medical Association, and the American Civil Liberties Union. The Appeals Court in Washington DC, heard the case and on 26th April 1990 it decided by seven to one that a pregnant woman may not be ordered to undergo a caesarean section to save her fetus [12].

Re S – an aberration?

Notwithstanding the legal position in the UK which accepts the autonomy of a lucid adult and accords the unborn child no rights independent of its mother, there was the case of *Re S* in October 1992 when an adult, lucid mother pregnant with her third child refused a caesarean section. The operation was considered necessary to save both her life and the baby's. Both she and her husband refused consent to the operation on religious grounds. The doctors at the hospital where she was admitted as an in-patient (having been in labour for more than 2 days) applied through the health authority for a declaration that the operation could be performed lawfully without the mother's consent. Most surprisingly but under great pressure, Sir Stephen Brown, the President of the Family Division, granted the declaration that in a situation in which the lives of mother and the unborn child would both be at risk if the operation were not performed it was open to the court to make a declaration that the operation could be performed notwithstanding the mother's refusal of consent. In the event, the baby died and the mother became extremely ill [13].

Although the decision in *Re S* appears understandable on its facts, with the President of the Family Division possibly unwilling to allow two young children to become motherless and also acting in the hope of saving the unborn child, it is plainly at odds with UK law and other authorities and cannot be regarded as in line with precedent or principle. It is notable that in its review of the right to consent and refuse treatment, the Law Commission document does not support this case and neither did the Court of Appeal or the House of Lords when reviewing the authorities in the case of *Airedale NHS Trust* v. *Bland* (1993) [14].

9.4.4 The basic dilemmas – (2) refusal of consent leading to death

Refusal not to be overriden

The courts have gone to some lengths to make it clear that where there is a validly given refusal, albeit that it seems unreasonable and not to be in the patient's interest as perceived by the providers of the health care including doctors and nurses in charge of the patient, this is not a reason to disregard it. The case of *Re T* (1992), in which an apparent refusal to treatment was overridden by a Court declaration, can be justified on the ground that T was under the undue influence of her mother when she refused blood transfusions and furthermore at the time (before she became unconscious) she had no idea of the seriousness of the consequences which would follow.

Indeed, the court considered the Canadian case of *Malette* v. *Shulman* (1990). This involved a Jehovah's Witness who carried a card stating that she did not wish to have blood administered in any circumstances. She was admitted to a casualty department following a very severe road accident in which her husband was killed. The casualty surgeon decided to provide blood transfusions notwithstanding the fact that he knew of the card and that she would have refused the treatment. Damages for battery were awarded. In the Court of Appeal decision in *Re T* (1992) [15] all three members of the Court of Appeal made it clear that a person in such circumstances was entitled to have his wishes respected.

Qualified refusal

However, Doctors and other health care providers must be sure that the refusal to treatment covers the particular situation. In *Malette* v. *Shulman* blood was not to be administered under *any* circumstances, but some refusals may be more limited in scope, perhaps applying 'so long as there is an effective alternative'.

Advance directives

In *Malette* v. *Shulman* the Ontario Court of Appeal made it clear that it was not concerned with

'A patient who has been diagnosed as terminally or incurably ill who seeks by way of advanced directive or "living will" to reject medical treatment so that she may die with dignity.'

However in a later case the same Court referred to the right to give binding advance directives as a 'traditional common law principle' [16].

In paragraph 3.7 of the Law Commission Paper [17], it is acknowledged that:

'In England and Wales, the dicta in *Re T*, together with those in *Airedale NHS Trust* v. *Bland* in both the Court of Appeal and the House of Lords indicate that an anticipatory decision which is "clearly established" and "applicable in the circumstances" may be as effective as the current decision of a capable adult.'

Since the case of S, there have been a number of other instances recorded in the general press of patients who refuse medical treatment on religious grounds being allowed to die.

9.5 Case study B – pain and the dying patient

Case B concerns a dying patient who is suffering great pain.

9.5.1 *The facts*

Mr B was a widower who lived alone and liked to be independent. He had enjoyed good health until he was diagnosed as suffering from cancer six months earlier. He had undergone sophisticated treatment in hospital including an operation and then radiotherapy which he had found distressing and unpleasant and his condition caused him considerable pain and left him weak and unable to do much more than potter about the house and struggle up to the shops once a week. A further visit to the hospital had revealed that the original tumour had not been completely excised and was beginning to spread and there were secondaries. The prognosis was extremely poor and he was not expected to live more than six to nine months during which his overall condition was likely to deteriorate. His married son lived in Scotland and could only visit occasionally and although neighbours did call round fairly regularly, he required district nursing services. He was under the care of his GP who was in contact with the specialist hospital concerned and who prescribed him painkilling drugs.

Gradually Mr B's condition deteriorated but he continued to refuse in-patient hospital admission or aggressive treatment for his cancer. As he grew weaker, he was unable to get to the shops, even accompanied, so that all his provisions had to be delivered or fetched by neighbours and the GP again pressed Mr B, as did the district nurse and the nurse sent from the general practice, that he should go into hospital where he could be properly cared for. Mr B refused, saying he wished to die in his own home, the sooner the better. Mr B was now requiring increasing amounts of morphine and the nurse who administered most of the injections which had been prescribed by the doctor became increasingly concerned that he was becoming addicted to morphine and she was also fearful that in a moment of despair he would try to take his own life. She felt the doctor was precribing too much morphine and did not always give the full amount recommended, as in her judgment it was more than required. Indeed she argued with the doctor about the quantities of morphine to be given making it clear she was unwilling to give such large quantities, fearing that the drug would shorten the patient's life and cause addiction.

Mr. B suffered considerable pain but again when pressed refused to be taken to hospital. The next day when the nurse called to check on his condition and give him a pain-killing injection he was found in a critical state. An empty bottle of paracetamol tablets was on the bedside table and he had left a short note apologising for 'letting them down', indicating that he intended to 'end my life before the cancer does', and begging anyone who found him still alive not to attempt resuscitation.

9.5.2 *Legal issues raised and steps to be taken*

Some of the same issues fall to be considered in this case as in that of Mrs A, though the circumstances are very different. Here the patient is making a value judgment on the quality of his life. He has formed the view that it is not worth preserving and indeed desirable that it should be ended prematurely.

Pain relief

While the nurse has a duty to use her professional judgment in providing medical care, it is submitted that she was not entitled to disregard the advice of the prescribing doctor whose qualifications are superior and reduce the dose of painkilling drugs simply out of fear that the patient would become addicted to them or that they could shorten his life. In the first place, dependence in such circumstances is of no matter since there is no long-term future lying ahead and the greatest concern must be to relieve pain. If this cannot be achieved without causing dependence then so be it. Unfortunately, in Britain, it seems that inadequate pain relief is commonly given when in fact this could be achieved.

In this case, it is uncertain whether it was the reduced dose of morphine and the failure to provide adequate pain relief that caused this patient to decide to take his own life at this time. In fact the likelihood is that at any future point he may have done so, but continued severe pain is extremely demoralizing and hard to bear, most particularly when no improvement is expected and indeed only deterioration is likely. Nurses should be careful to ensure that the pain relief that they are providing is *indeed* adequate and to alert the prescribing doctor if they feel that the pain relieving medication is not having the desired result.

The nurse who, 'off her own bat' in this way, tampers with the dose prescribed will expose herself to criticism and potential civil and perhaps disciplinary or even criminal proceedings if the outcome is bad.

Assessing the patient's state of mind

The nurse is the person who has the most regular contact with the patient for the most part and has an ideal opportunity to assess his progress and his state of mind and she should be alert to this. She should ensure that she is, and appears, accessible and approachable and that the patient has confidence in her. Very often, the nurse will be the first person in whom the patient will confide.

Steps to be taken

In this case, the patient has made it quite clear that he does not wish to have treatment to revive him and resuscitate him and that any such treatment provided would therefore prima facie be unlawful. However, it would be sensible for the nurse to telephone the patient's GP or other doctor in charge of his treatment and inform him of what has happened, and probably it would be appropriate for the patient to be removed to hospital albeit that no aggressive treatment aimed at resuscitation would be offered in the circumstances. However, if the patient has made it clear that he wishes to be left to die in his own home, then where possible this should be respected.

9.5.3 The basic dilemma – allowing death

Where the patient is critically ill but is no longer lucid, the decision as to whether or not to provide more than palliative care will lie with the doctor who should consult with the closest relatives or spouse wherever possible. However, the treatment he provides must be justifiable as in the patient's best interests. The best interest criteria set out in the Law Commission's Consultation Paper 129 (see Section 9.2.3) provide guidance on the factors which should be taken into account.

If the patient has expressed his wishes when lucid by means of an advance directive (although this is unlikely at present) or in the form of a letter written to his doctor or a statement in his will held by his solicitor or his next of kin, and this can be produced, this should assist in decision making. Wherever possible the patient's wishes should be respected.

Maintaining life

Where the patient is suffering from severe disability and is no longer mentally capable and, say, becomes ill with pneumonia, the question arises as to whether it is appropriate to treat with antibiotics or to allow the patient to die. Where the doctor is pressed by close relatives or a spouse to keep the patient alive and this is not contra-indicated by some form of advance directive, and can be justified as being in the patient's best interests, then this is probably the course that most doctors would take. However, there can be difficulties where relatives disagree and in the doctor's view the patient should be allowed to die. The doctor is unlikely to wish to become the focus of a dispute and it may well be easier to treat than allow the patient to die, even though that might be perceived as the better option. Palliative care should always be offered and the patient kept as comfortable as possible even if no aggressive therapeutic treatment is undertaken in the hope of improving the patient's overall prognosis.

Refusing care

Cases where patients or their families refuse treatment which their doctors consider to be in their best interests will always be difficult for the providers of medical care, most particularly nurses responsible for the day-to-day care of the patient. However, although this difficulty was recognized in the case of *Airedale NHS Trust* v. *Bland*, the House of Lords upheld the decision (unanimous with every judge who heard the arguments) that medical treatment including artificial hydration and nutrition, should be discontinued and the patient allowed to die in this way. However, the patient had absolutely no sensation of pain.

Palliative care or euthanasia?

It is difficult to justify in commonsense terms why it is lawful to discontinue treatment and allow the patient to die over a long period but not lawful to administer a lethal injection in such circumstances which would have a desired effect much more satisfactorily as was the case in *R* v. *Cox* (1993). However, while the law accepts that it is lawful to shorten life where the primary aim is to relieve pain *R* v. *Bodkin Adams* (1957), there is no provision for euthanasia or 'mercy killing' in English law and such acts aimed primarily at causing death are designated as homicide [17]. Nurses who suspect that such action has been taken are within their rights to report a doctor to the authorities (in both *Cox* and *R* v. *Arthur* (1981) it was a nurse who brought the case to the attention of the authorities) but many would not wish to do so though they may feel unhappy about sharing complicity in what they know to be contrary to the letter of the law and condoning an unlawful homicide, albeit for the best of motives. History makes it clear that the 'slippery slope' argument has considerable force justifying concern. Nurses should also be careful that they are not inveigled into assisting, aiding, abetting or procuring a suicide (contrary to the Suicide Act 1961) by fetching or administering bottles of tablets to patients who are too feeble to carry them for themselves.

The House of Lords Committee did not recommend legalizing euthanasia but with their endorsement there is little doubt that the future will see a development with regard to advance directives. It is important to ensure that patients should die as well as live with dignity.

9.6 Notes and references

1. See *R* v. *Secretary of State for Social Services, ex parte Hincks* (1970) 123 Sol Jo 436. See also Finch, J.D., *Health Services Law*, 1981: pp 38–9 and Brahams, D., 'Enforcing a duty to care for patients in the NHS.' *The Lancet*, 1984; ii; p 1224. Also *Re Walker's Application* (1987) *The Times*, 26 November (a Court of Appeal hearing on a baby's surgery being postponed five times due to shortage of skilled nursing staff) followed two months later by *R* v. *Central Birmingham Health Authority, ex parte Collier* (1988) *The Times* 6 January (against the same health authority), both cases discussed by Brahams, D. 'Seeking increased resources through the Courts.' *The Lancet* 1988; i; p 133.
2. Compare the discussion of the United States case of AC in Brahams, D. 'A baby's life or a mother's liberty.' *The Lancet* 1988; i; p 1006, Annas, G.J., 'She's going to die: the case of Angela C.' *Hastings Center Report*; February/March 1988; p 23, and Brahams, D. 'Enforced caesarean section: a US appeal.' *The Lancet* 1990; i; p 1270. See also 'Unwanted life

sustaining treatment.' The *Lancet* 1990; i, p 1209. Compare also the cases *Re T* (1992) and *Re S* (1992).

3. Considered in *F* v. *West Berkshire Health Authority* (1989) and approved in *Airedale NHS Trust* v. *Bland* (1993).

4. The Law Commission, *Mentally Incapacitated Adults and Decision-Making: Medical Treatment and Research* (Consultation Paper No. 129), London: HMSO, 1993.

5. The Law Commission, *Mentally Incapacitated Adults and Decision-Making: Medical Treatment and Research* (Consultation Paper No. 129), London: HMSO, 1993: part II paras 12 and 13. See also section 8.2.4 of this book.

6. For discussion, see Brahams, D., 'Criminality and Compassion.' *The Law Society's Gazette* 1992; 89/35; 30 September; p 2. For similar discussion of the *Airedale NHS Trust* v. *Bland* case while at Court of Appeal level, see Brahams, D., 'Of Life and Death.' *The Law Society's Gazette 1992*; 89/46; 16 December; p 3. For a discussion of the legal and ethical issues see also Mason, J.K., McCall Smith, A., *Law and Medical Ethics*, 4th edn., London: Butterworths, 1994 and Brazier, M., *Medicine, Patients and the Law*, 2nd edn., Harmondsworth: Penguin, 1992.

7. House of Lords, Paper 67, London: HMSO, 1993.

8. House of Lords, Paper 21, Vol I: Report VII: Oral evidence; Vol III: Written evidence. London: HMSO, 1994.

9. See Sheldon, A., 'Judges make historic ruling on euthanasia.' *British Medical Journal*; 309; p 7.

10. British Medical Association (Statement on Advance Directives) BMA, London, April 1993.

11. The Law Commission, *Mentally Incapacitated Adults and Decision-Making: Medical Treatment and Research* (Consultation Paper No. 129), London: HMSO, 1993: para 3.35.

12. For discussion in more detail of the case of *AC* see articles referred to in note 2 above and also Brahams, D. 'Fetus as Ward of Court' *The Lancet* 1988; i, p 369.

13. See also for discussion Brahams, D. 'Compulsory Intervention During Pregnancy.' *The Lancet* 1992; 340; p 1029. See also Re AC (1990) and Re T (1992).

14. For further discussion of the maternal-fetal conflict see Stein, E.J., Redman, C.W.G., 'Maternal-fetal Conflict: a Definition.' *Medico-legal Journal*; 58; 4; p 230.

15. Discussed Brahams, D., 'Right to Refuse Treatment.' *The Lancet* 1992; 340; p 297.

16. *Fleming* v. *Reid* 1991 82 DLR (4th) 298, 310. The case is cited at para 3.6 of the Law Commission Consultation Paper 129 (see below).

17. The Law Commission, *Mentally Incapacitated Adults and Decision-Making: Medical Treatment and Research* (Consultation Paper No. 129), London: HMSO, 1993: para 3.7.

18. See Devlin, P., *Easing the Passing, the Trial of Dr John Bodkin Adams*. Bodley Head, London, 1985. For an interesting discussion on the subject see Harvard, J.D., 'Aiding and Abetting suicides, the right to die and euthanasia. In (Brahams, D., ed) *Medicine and the Law*, Royal College of Physicians publications, 1990.

B An Ethical Perspective – Declining and Withdrawing Treatment
Robert Campbell

9.7 Introduction

How ought we to treat and care for patients who are dying? There are usually many things we can do but it is sometimes questionable whether they are all worth doing. For example, there was the case of

> ... a doctor aged sixty-eight dying of an inoperable cancer of the stomach. First it was treated by palliative removal of part of the stomach. Shortly afterwards the patient developed a pulmonary embolism and this was removed by an operation. Again he collapsed with myocardial infarction and was revived by the cardiac resuscitation team. His heart stopped on four subsequent occasions and was restarted artificially. The body lingered on for a few more weeks, with severe brain damage following the cardiac arrest and episodes of vomiting accompanied by generalized convulsions.
>
> This man had been told that he had stomach cancer; he accepted the diagnosis, which was confirmed by histological examination. Because the cancer had spread to his bones he suffered severe pain that was unrelieved by morphine or pethidine. When his pulmonary embolus was removed he was grateful, but asked that no further attempts should be made to resuscitate him should he require it. The request was not regarded [1].

Clearly the decision was made to attempt *every* possible procedure which could conceivably have prolonged the patient's life. In that sense, those procedures were worth attempting, because they did win him a few more weeks of life. There was, however, a cost. Not only did the patient suffer the pain and distress that the procedures themselves involved, but he was also subjected to the additional pain caused by the spreading cancer during those extra few weeks when he might, without such aggressive interventions, have died earlier. This cost was a high one and it seems worth asking whether the extra weeks of life were worth it. Compare that example with this one:

> A man in his late 50s had been in hospital for eight years on account of advanced Parkinson's disease. During the last year of his life he lost weight progressively, became generally weaker and spent more time in bed. He was less able to talk clearly and needed increasing help with the basic "activities of daily living". During this time he had three attacks of bronchitis. The first two were treated with chest physiotherapy and antibiotics. In anticipation of a further attack, it was decided that the man was in fact dying, albeit slowly, and that the next episode of bronchitis would not be treated with physiotherapy and antibiotics but simply symptomatically on the grounds that further curative treatment of the chest infection would, at this stage, be little more than "res-

urrecting the man to die again a few weeks later" or "prescribing a lingering death". The outcome of a chest infection in these circumstances was quite likely to be the man's death and it was seen as the natural terminal event of the progressive physical deterioration [2].

Here, by contrast, it might be asked whether the medical team accepted the situation and did what they could to ease the dying process or whether they gave up too readily. Indeed, in declining to offer further therapeutic treatment which might have extended the man's life, did they, in effect, operate a policy of passive euthanasia?

These are not purely medical questions. We are not asking what the limits of medical technology are, but rather how we decide when it is no longer consistent with the idea of giving the patient the best possible *care* to continue to attempt to *cure* him or her. These questions are inherently contestable and thus the patient's own views would be seen as authoritative as anyone else's views even if it were not the case that the importance of consent makes his or her views particularly crucial.

9.8 Why does consent matter?

The job of the nurses and other therapeutic team members is to do their best for the patient, given the resources at their disposal. Indeed, this is more than their job, it is their legal and moral duty once the patient has been accepted as a patient. It is hard to see how the patient, unless in some way deranged, can object to this. After all, is it not one of our informal tests for how sensible and rational someone is that they should want the best for themselves? Why should we also need their consent? There are three major reasons why we do.

9.8.1 *Persons of equal moral validity*

The first is located in the idea of a *person*. Most human beings are persons and most persons are human beings, but the terms do not have the same meaning [3]. A human being is a member of the biological species *homo sapiens*; a person is a moral agent who has plans and purposes and the capacity for free choice. From the point of view of personhood, all persons are morally equal in as much as there is no inherent reason for preferring one's plans and purposes to another's.

Disregarding a patient's right to consent to, or to refuse, treatment ignores the fact that the patient is an agent and assumes that your plan to treat a patient in a particular way is the only plan that matters. It is, in Kantian terminology, to treat the patient as a means to an end and not as an end-in-herself. It, therefore, fails to accord that patient the respect and dignity due to a person whose moral importance is as great as your own. If you believe that your plans and choices are important, then you must acknowledge that those of other persons are just as important. To fail to do so is a failure of logic as well as a failure of morality.

9.8.2 *Involvement in the treatment*

The second reason why consent matters has to do with human psychology rather than logic or morality. Patients whose agreement to treatment has been sought and obtained will feel empowered in a number of ways. Firstly they will *own* the treatment as an equal member of the team which has decided on it. They will be acting, rather than acted on. Secondly they will be less apprehensive about what will happen since, if the agreement is real and not just stage-managed, they will understand what is involved and its implications. Thirdly they will have retained control over their situation and, in situations where people are profoundly vulnerable and probably distressed, this is clearly, and in some cases literally, vital. They will feel, and be, *autonomous*. And since that term means no more than being a free moral agent, a person, this second point connects us back to the first again. It is also important to see that this process of empowerment will go on whether the patient agrees with the proposed course of treatment or whether they refuse it.

9.8.3 *Knowing what is best for oneself*

The third reason why consent matters has to do with what might be called fallibilism. People can be wrong and, in particular, they can be wrong about what is good for another person. The health care team is composed of experts in various fields, but the only person who is an expert on what is good for me is me. Admittedly the concept of fallibilism applies here too. I can be wrong about what is in my own best interests. We all know that can happen. But I am, normally, less likely to be wrong about it than someone else is and, in any case, if I am wrong I bear the consequences. So I have an incentive that they lack [4] to get it right. It is, therefore, vitally important when decisions need to be taken about what will be good for me, that I take them, even though I may need expert advice from others. What this means, in practice, is that I must have the opportunity to decide whether to accept the treatment offered, even though others may feel that my decision is the wrong one.

9.9 Refusing life-saving treatment

9.9.1 *Self-deterioration to the point of self-destruction*

From a philosophical point of view there is a troubling lack of symmetry between consenting to treatment on the one hand, and declining life-saving treatment on the other. For if the moral importance of consent is to be located in the idea of autonomy, i.e. self-determination, then choosing a course of action which you know is highly likely to result in your death seems inconsistent with this. Self-determination disappears when there is no self left to determine. Perhaps we can merely pass over this as a puzzling oddity since there are many other examples of it which we can accept quite readily:

- people who risk their lives, and lose them, in the attempt to help others;
- people who choose death rather than the violation of some principle or value which seems to them more important than their own lives [5]; and
- people who rationally choose to commit suicide.

Counselling this latter category does, however, raise some practical difficulties also thrown up in dealing with those who refuse life-saving treatment. For the general principle that people should make their own decisions and learn from their own mistakes cuts a little too deeply here. If choosing suicide or refusing treatment turns out to have been a mistake, then it is, in the nature of things, too late to learn anything from that. Just as consent can only be genuine if the patient fully understands what she is consenting to so, equally, the decision to refuse life-saving treatment should only be respected if it is clear that the patient understands the consequences of the refusal and also that the refusal is exactly what it seems to be.

9.9.2 *The pathological block*

Case Study A, as set out by Diana Brahams at section 9.5, seems to be such a case, but also cited frequently in this book is the case of *Re T* (1992) where the court decided that the refusal was made under the undue influence of the patient's mother and that there was reason to believe that the patient did not fully understand its implications. There might be enormous difficulty in determining this kind of issue. In the American case, *State of Tennessee Department of Human Services* v. *Mary C. Northern* (1978) [6], was described by the guardian appointed for her by the court as '72 years of age . . . in possession of a good memory and recall, respond[ing] accurately to questions asked her . . . coherent and intelligent in her conversation and . . . of sound mind.' She was suffering from gangrene in both feet consequent upon frostbite and burns, but refused to have the feet amputated, as her surgeons were urging her to do. Though otherwise apparently entirely rational, it emerged in conversation that she very much wanted to live *and* very much wanted to save her feet. She did not seem able to grasp that there

was only a one in ten chance that both things could happen and reso-
lutely refused to consider, except as an abstract hypothesis, that she
would have to choose between them. The court decided to authorize
surgery, apparently accepting the view that an otherwise competent
adult might, nonetheless, be incompetent in the matter of one specific
decision. In the light of the transcripts, which are too lengthy to quote
here, this would seem to have been the morally right decision. Mary
Northern seems to have combined a general rational competence with a
pathological block with regard to the condition of her feet, which she
believed had got better and about which her physicians were lying or
mistaken.

9.9.3   An external system of belief

How are we to align the lesson of this case with Case Study A? May we
characterize Jehovah's Witnesses as otherwise rational patients with a
pathological block about blood transfusions? We might wish to argue
that Jehovah's Witnesses are not irrational, they simply have beliefs
which the rest of us do not share but cannot disprove. But Mary
Northern's irrationality, in the end, came down to her refusal to give up
a belief about the condition of her feet which no one was able to prove
to her was false. There is no easy answer to the question of what makes
belief irrational. It may help to resolve the problem of distinguishing the
beliefs of Jehovah's Witnesses from those of people like Mary Northern
to note that Mary Northern's beliefs came from nowhere, that they were
ungrounded by anything apart from what seems to be a desperate
attempt to wish the circumstances other than they actually were. The
beliefs of Jehovah's Witnesses do form a system, they are shared by
large numbers of people and they are culturally transmitted – they have
rational validation even if not by those who are not Jehovah's
Witnesses. This is hardly conclusive, but it is persuasive.

9.10   Balancing rights

There is another factor, however, in Case Study A which is disquieting.
The mother's refusal of treatment did not just involve herself, but her
unborn baby. The law may not recognize the rights of an unborn child,
but from a moral point of view it would be curious to assert that a fetus at
term is, in itself, in any significant way different from a new born baby.
What might be arguable is whether its life may be saved at the cost of
what has been called a 'massive intrusion into a person's body' [7], i.e. a
caesarean section. In a parallel American case, that of Angela Carder
[8], the original decision to permit the caesarean section was voided on
appeal and Angela Carder's parents won undisclosed damages from the

hospital in a separate action for medical malpractice, wrongful death and violation of civil rights. In that case neither the mother nor the child survived the operation. Though the mother was suffering widespread and irreversible cancer of the bone and lungs, the death certificate listed the caesarean as a contributing factor.

A caesarean section is a major surgical intervention, with all the risks and dangers that this involves. It would seem unreasonable to *require* someone to take those risks in order to benefit someone else. In another American case, the courts ruled that someone cannot be forced to donate bone-marrow (a procedure considerably less risky than a caesarean section) even where failure to do so would result in the death of a third party (because only one person could be found who was tissue-type compatible) [9]. But it does not follow that that person had no *moral* obligation to be a bone-marrow donor, nor that we may not think badly of him for ducking it. Nor is there an exact carry-over from that case to Case Study A. It is arguable that those who willingly become pregnant have, in doing so, already accepted a degree of moral responsibility for the welfare of the child they carry. In addition a caesarean section is not so dangerous or unusual an intervention that it is obvious that no one could be expected to risk it. Nor are the declared grounds for refusal as coherent as they may seem. According to *The Guardian*, Jehovah's Witnesses do not normally object to caesarean sections as a matter of principle providing they do not involve blood transfusions [10].

Here there is clearly a balance to be struck between anyone's right to refuse life-saving treatment and the rights of the unborn child (which must have some moral force even if not normally recognized in English law). There must also be a question mark, though perhaps not more than that, over the coherence of the reasons given. These considerations ought to affect what happens when treatment is refused, or indications are given that it will be. Efforts should be made to explain the consequences of the refusal and to persuade the patient to reconsider. It would be desirable, in such a case, to ask for the patient's spiritual adviser to offer counselling. If the patient is simply mistaken about what his or her religious beliefs require, then the situation could be resolved at this stage.

Though there are good moral reasons to criticize or even oppose some decisions to refuse life-saving treatment, it may well be that there are equally good policy reasons for not giving that opposition legal force. We may, in other words, disagree, perhaps profoundly, with a decision without thinking that it would be right to enforce another course of action on the patient. Clearly, for example, there are excellent reasons for thinking that a general policy of enforcing caesarean sections on unwilling women would be an extremely bad thing.

9.11 Withdrawing treatment

9.11.1 *The moral view*

In the introduction I mentioned the case of a patient from whom treatment was withdrawn on the grounds that he was, in fact, dying and it was considered neither proper nor humane simply to prolong the dying process. Both the American and British Medical Associations endorse this view, as do the Catholic and Anglican Churches:

> 'The cessation of the employment of extraordinary means to prolong the life of the body when there is irrefutable evidence that biological death is imminent is the decision of the patient and/or his immediate family' [11].

> 'In its narrow current sense, euthanasia implies killing, and it is misleading to extend it to cover decisions not to preserve life by artificial means when it would be better for the patient to be allowed to die. Such decisions coupled with a determination to give the patient as good a death as possible, may be quite legitimate' [12].

> '... normally one is held to use ordinary means ... that is to say, means that do not involve any grave burden for oneself or another.... Consequently, if it appears that the attempt at resuscitation constitutes such a burden for the family that one cannot in all conscience impose it upon them, they can lawfully insist that the doctor should discontinue those attempts and the doctor can lawfully comply' [13].

> 'The distinction between deliberate killing and the administration of painkilling drugs or the withdrawal of treatment such as to have the effect of shortening life, though sometimes a very fine one in practice, must remain a guiding principle' [14].

It is widely believed that this position involves drawing a moral distinction between active and passive euthanasia. Some people, perhaps most people, seem to think that if euthanasia can be justified at all, it can be justified more readily if it is passive rather than active. In what follows I consider the ethical issues behind the cases of *Bland* and *Cox*. This will indicate the complexity of these issues and show why placing so much emphasis on the distinction between active and passive euthanasia is misleading.

9.11.2 *Tony Bland*

Tony Bland was a victim of the Hillsborough football disaster. As a result of his injuries he was comatose and remained in a persistent vegetative state until 1993 when his parents applied through the courts for permission for artificial nutrition and hydration to be withdrawn, and for antibiotics not to be given. The courts held that artificial nutrition and hydration was a form of treatment. They also held that because Mr Bland would not recover, the treatment was of no benefit to him, and withdrawing it would take the form of a legal omission rather than commission, i.e. the medical team had no duty to continue to treat Mr Bland.

The arguments were:

(1) A doctor is under no duty to continue to treat a patient where such treatment confers no benefit on the patient.
(2) Being maintained in a persistent vegetative state with no prospect of recovery was regarded by informed medical opinion as not being a benefit to a patient.
(3) The principle of the sanctity of life was not absolute, for example
   - where a patient expressly refuses treatment, even though death may well be a consequence of that refusal,
   - where a prisoner on hunger strike refuses food and may not be forcibly fed,
   - where a patient is terminally ill, death is imminent and treatment will only prolong suffering.
(4) Artificial hydration and nutrition required medical intervention for its application and was widely regarded by the medical profession as medical treatment.

It is clear, therefore, that the governing principle here was not that it was permissible to let a patient die so long as he or she was not actually *killed*; rather that *caring* for a patient (in cases where cure was not possible and recovery was extremely unlikely) did not require medical interventions which were of no benefit to the patient. Nonetheless, it is also arguable that the treatment in question was not a *disbenefit* to Bland; if it did him no good, it also did him no harm. If doctors were under no duty to treat Bland, they were also under no duty not to. But discontinuing treatment was a benefit – to Bland's relatives and friends, especially his parents, who were to be spared the grief of continuing to see their son in this exceptionally distressing condition and would, finally, be able to mourn the loss they had suffered two years before. That is far from a negligible benefit and if, whatever happened, nothing more could be done to harm or benefit Bland himself, it seems right to let the choice of outcome be decided by what would most benefit those closest to him.

9.11.3 *Dr Nigel Cox*

It is interesting to compare the circumstances of Tony Bland with these of Lilian Boyes. Dr Nigel Cox was found guilty of attempted murder in 1992 for administering a lethal dose of potassium chloride to a patient, Lilian Boyes, who, dying and in acute pain, had pleaded with him to help her die. It is hard to see how, on the face of it, this case is to be distinguished from that of *Bland*, without invoking the distinction between active and passive euthanasia. The remarks of Dame Elizabeth Butler-Sloss, Lord Justice in the Court of Appeal hearing of *Bland* would seem to do just that.

> 'The position of Dr Nigel Cox, who injected a lethal dose designed to cause death, was different since it was an external and intrusive act and was not in accordance with his duty of care as a doctor. The distinction between Mr Bland's doctors and Dr Cox was between an act or omission which allowed causes already present in the body to operate and the introduction of an external agency of death.'

The Guardian's leader writer called that position a 'philosophical nonsense,' [15] and maybe it is, if taken at face value. However, there are other morally relevant distinctions to be drawn between the two cases [16] If we were to say that Dr Cox's decision was the morally right one in the circumstances then the explanation for its rightness must be different from the explanation of the rightness of withdrawing treatment from Tony Bland.

9.11.4   *The principle of double effect*

The source of this distinction is an old notion thought by many to be now discredited called 'the principle of double effect'. It should, I think, be seen not as a rule for resolving moral problems but as a guide which can clarify what is at issue in particular cases. It relies on a distinction between what one intends and what one merely foresees as a result of one's actions. The principle suggests that, whereas one is fully responsible for what one intends to do, one is not responsible for foreseen but unintended effects of one's actions, provided that:

(1) What is done must be, at the least, morally permissible.
(2) What is intended must include only the good and not the bad effects of what is done.
(3) The bad effects must not be the *means* whereby the good is brought about.
(4) There must be *proportionality* between the good and bad effects of what is done.

Thus the distinction which I am suggesting matters between *Cox* and

Bland is that, whereas Dr Cox must have intended Lilian Boyes' death as the only way as he saw it of sparing her further pain and suffering, Tony Bland's medical team intended to spare him further treatment whilst foreseeing that this would probably lead to his death. This distinction may have no practical force in those two actual cases, but it matters to the extent that we are prepared to generalize from them.

I do not believe that passive euthanasia is permissible because it is merely a matter of allowing patients to die rather than acting in order to bring about their death. But I do believe that in cases where the patient's death is imminent, or where treatment is painful and offers only a very remote chance of success, then it is justifiable (if the patient and/or her relatives consent) to cease to continue treatment. In the case of Tony Bland, the only effect that continuing his treatment could have had would have been to postpone the date of his death, together with the perpetuation of the distress and grief caused to his parents and relatives.

Moral responsibility for an event is not determined by whether it came about because one acted or failed to act; it is determined by one's intentions and duties. If there is no duty, moral or legal, to treat, and also persuasive reasons for not doing so, it must normally be entirely permissible to withdraw treatment, even if to do so results in the death of the patient.

The case of *Cox* is different. Far from discontinuing pointless treatment, he was forced, as he saw it, to treat his patient so that she would die. He both had, and recognized by his actions, a continuing duty to treat. Whether that kind of treatment can be morally justified depends on whether any available option would have been preferable. What can be said is that it is possible to imagine circumstances where the suffering of the patient is so great and the possibility of immediate remedy so small that killing the patient is the only available means of preventing the pain. In national disasters or wars such circumstances may arise, or in parts of the world where medical resources are extremely limited. In those circumstances it is arguable that acting so as to bring about the death of the patient as easily and quickly as possible might not be wrong [17]. It may be that the circumstances in which Nigel Cox found himself were equivalent to these, in which case, he has that justification. Only those involved are well placed to make this judgment, and for that reason we cannot say conclusively that what Dr Cox did was wrong; but, also for that reason, it is an option which, on policy grounds and in general, it would be unwise for the law to sanction.

9.12 Caring and curing

I mentioned earlier the tension that can exist between curative treatment and care; when persisting with attempts to cure may no longer be consistent with providing the best possible care for the patient. This will be a problem when caring is *identified* with curing and so the attempt to cure is continued long after it has ceased to be appropriate in the mistaken belief that not to do so would be to cease to care for the patient. Case Study B also demonstrates the dangers of identifying too closely care and cure. Mr B resists the therapeutic options he is offered, as is his right, but he thereby leaves the health care team dealing with his case apparently at a virtual loss as to what more they can do. Morphine alone is prescribed for pain-relief and even this is under-mined by his nurse's misplaced anxieties concerning possible addiction.

We need not doubt the health care team's motivation or sincerity in order to question whether this amounted to appropriate care for Mr B. Care requires resources just as much as therapy does. The resources lacking here would seem to be training in and information about the care of the terminally ill and, in particular, ways of dealing with chronic physical pain and emotional distress. One of the valuable things to be learnt from the experience of the hospice movement is that the final stages of a terminal illness, even a difficult one like cancer, need not be like Mr B's. It is pain, fear and despair which leads most terminally ill patients to attempt suicide or ask for euthanasia. In the hospice, it is precisely those factors which are addressed, through specialist pain control and counselling [18]. Once in control of their pain and themselves, it is often found that patients are able to order their lives and prepare for their death.

Mr B received little or no counselling specific to his situation and his pain was poorly controlled. It seems that the apparent dilemma – whether to accept his decision to refuse treatment or simply to override it – is a bogus one, and alternatives were available which might have made it possible for him to defer his decision 'to end my life before the cancer does' a little longer. We do not know whether these alternatives – access to a hospice or a specialist Macmillan nurse – were available to the practice treating Mr B, but it is quite possible they were not. The present NHS arrangements mean that they are available when charitable donations permit but not otherwise. The resourcing of the system is skewed towards the scientific war on disease and illness in terms of cure. Prevention and care are thought of as secondary when they are remembered at all. Mr B could not have been *cured*, but he might have been better *cared* for.

9.13 Notes and references

1. Gresham, G.A. 'A Time to be Born and a Time to Die', in Downing, A.B., ed. *Euthanasia and the Right to Death*. London: Peter Owen, 1969: p 150. See also Symmers, W.St.C. Sr., 'Not Allowed to Die', *British Medical Journal*, 1 (1986), 442.

2. The Linacre Centre *Euthanasia and Clinical Practice*, 1982: p 57.

3. For example, it has been doubted whether babies, fetuses, or those who, whilst still biologically alive, lack any response to the world around them are persons in the strict sense of the term. (See Weir, R.F. *Abating Treatment with Critically Ill Patients* New York: Oxford University Press, 1989; pp 70–71 and 405–412.) It can also be argued that higher apes and cetaceans (dolphins, porpoises and whales) might conceivably be persons in the required sense. (See Singer, P. *Practical Ethics*, Cambridge: Cambridge University Press, 1979.)

4. For a more complete, and classic, exposition of this view, see John Stuart Mill, *On Liberty*. (There are many editions of this, but a good recent one which includes critical essays is edited by John Gray and G.W. Smith (1991), *J.S. Mill On Liberty In Focus*, Routledge.)

5. For example, Thomas More (as described in *A Man For All Seasons*, by Robert Bolt), or John Proctor in Arthur Miller's *The Crucible*.

6. Cited in Arras J., & Rhoden, N. eds. *Ethical Issues in Modern Medicine*. 3rd edn., 1989: pp 72–9.

7. Judge John Terry, in the case of Angela Carder (district of Columbia Court of Appeals, 1990), the American case cited in evidence in *Re S*.

8. See further note 2 to section 9.6.

9. See *The Montreal Gazette*, 27 July 1978; the case is discussed in Campbell, R. Collinson, D. *Ending Lives*, Oxford: Blackwell Science Ltd 1988: pp 174–175.

10. See *The Guardian*, 14 July 1993, p 3.

11. *Journal of the American Medical Association*. 1974, p 227. See also the British Medical Association, *The Handbook of Medical Ethics*, London: BMA, 1981.

12. Church of England National Assembly Board for Social Responsibility. *On Dying Well*, London: Church Information Office, 1975; p 10. and *The Guardian* Leading article, 20 November 1992.

13. Pope Pius XII, *The Pope Speaks*, 4, no. 4, p 396.

14. Principles endorsed by the House of Bishops of the Church of England in October 1992, as cited by David Sheppard in a letter to *The Guardian*, 27 October 1992

15. *The Guardian* Leading article, 20 November 1992.

16. What follows should not be seen as implying any criticism of Dr Cox who, it would seem, was placed in an extremely difficult situation and, in all good faith, was doing what he believed was the only thing he could do to help Ms Boyes.

17. See Church of England National Assembly Board for Social Responsibility. *On Dying Well*, London: Church Information Office, 1975; p 10.

18. 'The "hospice concept" describes a number of areas of care of terminally ill patients and their families, which may be listed as: symptom control, effective communication, family support (including bereavement care), spiritual care, staff support, teaching and research'. Taken from Kearney, M. 'Hospice Medicine', in Seedhouse, D. Cribb A, eds *Changing Ideas in Health Care*. Chichester John Wiley and Sons, 1989; see also Laverton, R. *Care of the Dying*, Harmondsworth: Penguin, 1980.

Chapter 10
Research and Patients

A The Legal Perspective
Erika Kirk

10.1 Introduction

Biomedical research involving patients is a subject in which the disciplines of nursing, law, and ethics overlap in a particularly complex way. It is a subject which can attract adverse comment when problems emerge and patients are thought to be at risk; and yet without it advances in medicine and nursing care are not possible. It is therefore a subject which raises numerous questions about the legality and morality of conducting experiments on human beings.

It is not the aim of this part of the chapter to provide definitive answers to any of these questions. Instead this section attempts to provide a framework within which the main legal and ethical issues might be examined. It is hoped that this will enable health care professionals involved in research to make informed choices about their participation in such projects, and to appreciate any potential liability they may incur.

To begin with, it is worth considering what is meant by the terms 'research' and 'patients' for the purposes of this chapter.

10.1.1 Patients

A proportion of health care research is conducted with the good-will of healthy volunteers who have been recruited from the general population and who are willing to undergo some procedure in order to further the knowledge of nurses and other professionals. These healthy volunteers cannot be called patients in the true sense of the word. Similarly, research projects may involve the use of fetuses and fetal tissue, but again, this could not be described as research involving patients.

These two categories of research subject are not therefore included in the discussion of the law which follows. It is worth noting, however, that the legal provisions applicable to the use of healthy volunteers and to fetal material are substantially the same as those applicable to patients. The distinction between these groups is necessary, however, because of the greatly differing ethical considerations attaching to them.

The patients with whom this chapter is primarily concerned therefore are those who have consulted a doctor and who have as a result come within the normal therapeutic nurse/patient relationship, either in the primary health care sector or in hospital. Alternatively they may have been selected from the general population because of known or suspected abnormality [1].

10.1.2 *Research*

The definition of 'research' presents greater difficulties; in reality, the distinction between medical or nursing practice, innovative treatment (or experimentation), and research can be blurred, and on occasions all three activities may be occurring simultaneously. The Royal College of Physicians has distinguished between medical practice and medical research on the basis of intent [2]. In medical practice, the sole intention is to benefit the individual patient. In research, the primary intention is to advance knowledge so that patients in general may benefit. Thus, if the **prime** purpose of treating the patient is to make a systematic investigation to establish facts or to test a hypothesis and draw generalizable conclusions, that is research, even if some benefit does accrue to the patient as a result [3].

It will be clear to those involved in the care of patients, however, that in practice this distinction is not always so clear cut; and it makes no provision for the situation where a practitioner steps outside what is regarded as standard or accepted practice in an attempt to provide the best possible treatment for the benefit of a particular patient. Such a situation would seem to come within the definition of innovative treatment, or even an experiment i.e. a procedure adopted on the chance of its succeeding [4]. It would not seem to constitute research within the definition provided.

10.1.3 *Types of research*

From a nursing point of view, research in patients can thus be identified according to the prevailing intention of those carrying out the procedures involved. But that research can be further classified or categorised according to its aims. For example the aims and objectives of the procedure might be to investigate the causes of disease; to improve the diagnosis of disease; to improve the treatment and care of those suffering from disease; or to investigate the functioning of the human body. Whilst the particular aims of a research project may be an influential factor in determining its legality or its ethical status, even more important are the distinctions drawn concerning the methodology employed and the benefit (or lack of it) to the research subject. Thus significant legal and ethical questions will arise according to whether the research is

non-intrusive or **intrusive** vis-à-vis the subject, and whether it is **therapeutic** or **non-therapeutic** research [5].

- **Non-intrusive** research does not involve direct interference with the subject. It may involve making observations or an epidemiological study from medical records, but it does not directly impinge on the patient's mind or body.

- **Intrusive** research entails direct involvement with the subject. This may be non-invasive e.g. psychological inquiries or it may involve physical invasion e.g. surgical intervention.

- **Therapeutic** or clinical research involves research combined with professional care and is conducted with a view to benefitting the patients on whom it is carried out.

- **Non-therapeutic** or non-clinical research is a 'purely scientific application of medical research carried out on a human being' [6]. It involves volunteers who will not or who are unlikely to be benefited by the procedures, but who will provide the opportunity to further scientific knowledge. These volunteers may include patients who have no connection with the illness or process concerned, and healthy volunteers, e.g. students, or the researchers themselves, who are recruited to participate in the study.

These distinctions make a valuable contribution to any discussion of the legal and ethical basis for research in patients. For it becomes apparent that non-intrusive research will generally raise fewer legal and ethical problems than intrusive research; and that the greater the invasive or intrusive nature of the procedures, the more serious the ethical questions and potential legal problems. But it has been pointed out that these definitions carry their own dangers; particularly the possibility that 'any research on children and adults is acceptable so long as one can call it therapeutic research' [7].

It is also interesting to note that in determining the legal duty of care owed by nurses or doctors to their patients, the courts have declared that any distinction between advice given in a therapeutic context and in a non-therapeutic context is 'unwarranted and artificial'. (*Gold* v. *Harringey Health Authority* (1988)). There is no doubt however that these definitions are found useful in practice, and form the basis of professional guidelines on this subject [8].

10.1.4   *Legal control and ethical review*

Progress in the diagnosis and care of the sick depends upon research, and hospitals and community health care units are increasingly research-oriented. Indeed, the maintenance and improvement of professional knowledge and competence envisaged by the UKCC Code of Conduct [9] will depend in part on the advances in caring made through research. It is therefore important for all members of health care teams to be aware of their potential legal liabilities when research involving patients is conducted. It is equally important that research should be ethically acceptable to those carrying it out, to those who are the subjects of research, and to society in general. These issues will be considered in the second part of this chapter.

The remainder of this part of this chapter comprises an examination of the legal and quasi-legal issues, together with an illustrative case study.

10.2 Legal controls over research

Research involving patients of the type described in the case study which follows can have obvious benefits for the patients involved. Therefore, although it is intrusive in nature and carries some risk, it is yet therapeutic research, and its legality and its ethical status must be judged accordingly. From a legal point of view this type of research can be controlled by the relevant civil or criminal laws, breach of which will give rise to legal sanctions. Yet there is very little case or statute law which directly addresses the legal liability which researchers may incur when using patients as subjects. There are few legal rules formulated to deal specifically with research. Thus it is the general principles of civil and criminal law discussed here and elsewhere in this book which provide a framework for the regulation of research involving patients.

10.2.1 *The civil law*

If a person is subjected to some medical procedure which involves contact with that person's body, then, unless consent to that contact is freely given, the tort (legal wrong) of battery is committed. The person making that contact, whether doctor or nurse, in circumstances where no agreement has been given, is liable in damages simply because the patient has not authorized the touching. Thus where any research involves examining, operating upon or injecting the patient, consent must be obtained in advance if the research is to be carried out legally. For this consent to be real, the practitioner must explain the general nature of the procedure to the patient (*Chatterton* v. *Gerson* (1981) and must explain that the patient is involved in a research project. Where a practitioner is both caring for the patient and conducting research, the patient's consent is only genuine if the patient is aware of this dual intention [10].

Another tort which may arise out of research involving patients is that of negligence. If a piece of medical research is carried out in such a way that the researcher is in breach of the duty of care owed to a patient, then an action for negligence may ensue. In therapeutic research, where the researcher is responsible for the patient's care, as well as for the research, this duty of care is not hard to establish. Thus, use of a clearly inappropriate drug or an inappropriate amount of a drug would be obvious examples of negligence.

Negligence may also arise if there is a failure to obtain from the patient what is often referred to as 'informed consent'. Where the patient's treatment is determined on the basis of a research project, that patient's consent must be sought as to the treatment involved. To be fully effective, that consent must be based on a knowledge and under-standing of the procedures to be used and of the risks and side effects of treatment. This raises particular problems if the research is based on a complex scientific hypothesis, for this leads to the question of how such knowledge and understanding can be achieved, and how much infor-mation should be given to the patient in such circumstances. The answer is provided by the general law of negligence, for the '*Bolam test*' applies as much in research as it does in general health care practice.

The standard is set by a practitioner having that degree of compe-tence expected of the ordinary skilled practitioner. If the ordinary skilled practitioner, applying proper medical practice in accordance with a responsible body of medical opinion, would have carried out the research in a particular way, seeking the patient's consent in certain terms, then if the researcher fails to match these standards, an action for negligence may result. There may, however, be several 'approved' schools of practice which are deemed to be reasonable and the courts will not necessarily choose between them. This applies with equal force to the issue of warnings as to risks and side effects. If proper medical practice would require a patient in a clinical trial to be warned of the possibility of certain adverse reactions and risks of treatment, then that information must be given, or again liability in negligence may follow.

This latter point has particular application when considering the accountability of the nurse-practitioner. Frequently patients will request a nurse, rather than a doctor, to explain aspects of their treatment or care, or as in this case study, the research project. If the nurse does not feel that the patient has been given sufficient information in terms that the patient can readily understand, then the UKCC advisory document *Exercising Accountability* places a responsibility on the nurse to state this opinion and to seek to have the situation remedied. Indeed if the nurse is not convinced that the patient has given truly informed consent, then the nurse may decide not to co-operate with the procedure [11].

The issue of consent becomes particularly difficult when the subject of the medical research is a child, or any other person about whose capacity to give valid consent there is some doubt. These difficulties are referred to later in sections 10.5.2 and 10.5.3. Similarly, the question of consent to participation in randomized controlled trials can give rise to problems for the patient in consenting to what must remain an unknown treatment, a form of Russian roulette. Again this is an issue which is dealt with in greater depth in section 10.6.

To complete the picture, in terms of the civil law, liability could conceivably arise in circumstances where the relationship between researcher and patient was based on a contract. For example, if the patient was being treated in a private hospital and paying for drugs and medical care, liability for breach of contract would ensue if the researcher failed in some way to abide by the terms of the contract. This is however a far less common scenario than that envisaged by the case study.

10.2.2 *Criminal law*

The general criminal law applies to health care research and renders a member of the health care team liable to prosecution if an offence is committed. The most likely offences here would be assault (where a person fears that unlawful force is about to be applied to his body) and battery (where the unlawful force is actually carried out). For example, taking a blood sample without consent would be classed as a battery, and the apprehension that this about to occur as assault. Clearly there are exceptional situations, such as medical emergencies, where such a course of action may be necessary without obtaining prior consent. If the situation came within the established exceptions to the requirement of consent then no criminal prosecution would follow. Such exceptions are however of far more obvious application in general medical practice than in research; and thus consent remains of prime importance when carrying out invasive procedures for the purposes of research.

A less obvious but more likely way in which a breach of the criminal law might occur concerns compliance with the Medicines Act 1968. Medicinal products used in the UK generally require a product licence from the licensing authority i.e. UK Health and Agriculture Ministers. When an unlicensed product is to be used in clinical trials, then the supplier may be required to obtain a clinical trial certificate from the authority, permitting the use of the product. This requirement is waived, however, under what is known as the DDX provision, where the trial is being conducted by a doctor who takes responsibility for the research and initiates it, and where the doctor abides by certain conditions. Failure to observe these rules concerning the use of unlicensed products in clinical trials involving patients may lead to sanctions under the Act.

From the foregoing discussion, it appears that the crucial concept so far as **legal** control over research involving patients is concerned, is the concept of consent. Before this concept is examined in greater detail, however, it is useful to consider what might be called **non-legal** control of research i.e. the guidelines and codes of practice which do not directly have the force of law.

10.3 Non-legal controls over research

The threat of legal sanction if medical research is carried out negligently or without the requisite consents is a very real constraint on research. But equally real are the constraints which arise from professional declarations, codes of conduct, and from the work of Research Ethics Committees. Whilst not of themselves rendering researchers legally liable if breaches of these provisions occur, their influence pervades and restrains research, and breach of such codes may be used as an indicator of negligence in the researcher.

10.3.1 *Nuremberg Code and Declaration of Helsinki*

The first internationally recognized principles concerning biomedical research were published in 1949 in the Nuremberg Code. This document attempted to set the legal and moral boundaries for activities of this nature, in the wake of the medical experiments involving humans conducted during the Nazi régime. This was followed in 1964 by the Declaration of Helsinki which contains the recommendations of the World Medical Assembly, and which is periodically reviewed, most recently in 1989. Both the Code and the Declaration recognize the value and purpose of research involving human beings, but attempt to define 'certain basic principles which must be observed in order to satisfy moral, ethical and legal concepts' [12].

At the simplest level, these principles establish that the voluntary consent of the subject is essential, and that all unnecessary pain and suffering should be avoided. But at a more sophisticated level, the Declaration of Helsinki draws the distinction (already noted above) between therapeutic or clinical research, and non-therapeutic research, and highlights slightly different factors to be taken into account in each case [13]. It is from this Declaration that the requirement comes for procedures to be formulated in an experimental protocol and submitted to a specially appointed independent committee for consideration. It is here, too, that the so-called 'risk/benefit' test has its origins. This requires that any research project involving human subjects be preceded by a careful assessment of 'predictable risks in comparison with foreseeable benefits'.

10.3.2 *Professional guidelines*

Although the documents mentioned above form the very foundations for rules concerning the conduct of medical research, like many international codes they do not have the force of law. However it is possible to see how these principles have developed into the professional codes of conduct with which practitioners in the UK will be more familiar: the Royal College of Physicians has produced three reports, as a result of the deliberations of two working parties and of the College Committee on Ethical Issues in Medicine [14]. Similarly, the Royal College of Nursing has produced guidance for nurses involved in research projects [15]. It cannot be said that breach of the guidelines contained in these reports results in breach of any law (no civil or criminal liability is directly linked to these codes) and yet this professional guidance may prove to be the most influential factor in the conduct of research involving patients. These documents provide a source of information, opinion and guidance to all health care workers involved in research. Much of what is recommended might be regarded as the best practice in the field, and could form the standard against which the conduct of research could be judged in negligence cases. These are, therefore, guidelines which researchers ignore at their peril.

All three reports provide a useful discussion of the arguments concerning the ethical aspects of clinical and non-clinical trials, and elaborate on the general advice provided by the Nuremberg Code and the Declaration of Helsinki. They also make specific recommendations about such matters as obtaining consent, selecting and recruiting patients, and assessing the quality of research. Where the general law provides no guidance, these reports suggest ways to initiate and execute research in order to remain within the civil and criminal law, and to be aware of ethical issues. As such they are invaluable.

10.3.3 *Research ethics committees*

A further non-legal control over the work of researchers is found in the Research Ethics Committees. Little known by those outside the health care professions until relatively recently, these bodies have been established within the NHS since 1967 to be custodians of good practice in medical research. The objectives of Research Ethics Committees are [16]

- to maintain ethical standards of practice in research,
- to protect subjects of research from harm,
- to preserve the subjects' rights and
- to provide reassurance to the public that this is being done.

But the law provides no mandatory requirement that research projects be submitted for scrutiny – nor are there any legal sanctions if research is carried out without the approval of such a committee. Indeed the very existence of Ethics Committees is on an entirely non-legal basis, and research into the constitition, membership, and conduct of these committees has highlighted the lack of adequate control and supervision in this area [17].

The most important constraint here would appear to be professional peer pressure. The British Medical Association has stated that all clinical trials should be approved by a properly constituted ethics committee [18], and the Medical Research Council, and other bodies which fund research, require ethical review of projects prior to making a grant; some scientific journals require it as a condition of publication. These, then, are the influences which will encourage researchers to submit their work for independent review, rather than any fear of legal sanction.

10.4 Case study – Richard Douglas

Richard Douglas, a 15-year old boy of average intelligence, had suffered repeated chest infections from childhood. By his fifteenth birthday, this had developed into frequent bouts of wheezy bronchitis, and his GP referred him to a consultant at the local teaching hospital with suspected asthma.

The consultant to whom Richard was referred was engaged in a research project (approved by the Hospital Ethics Committee) into the treatment of childhood onset asthma. The project involved a controlled double blind clinical trial. Suitable patients were randomly placed in two groups. One group received a standard dosage of a drug of established efficacy delivered by inhaler, plus a placebo in tablet form. The other group received the same standard medication by inhaler but also received a multi-vitamin supplement in tablet form, containing a high dosage of vitamin B6. Possible side effects envisaged from the use of the multi-vitamin supplement were stomach upsets, skin rash, and pins and needles in the hands and feet. The trial was constructed in such a way that the doctor who would assess the progress of the patients was also blind to the identity of the trial treatment.

On Richard's second visit to the hospital, the consultant interviewed Richard with his mother Jane, and raised the possibility of entering him in the trial. At that point, Richard's younger brother felt sick, and Mrs Douglas had to escort him from the consulting room. In her absence, the consultant explained that Richard could be 'really helpful' by taking some 'new treatment'. He said that this would involve continued use of the inhaler to which Richard was now accustomed, but that there would also be an extra tablet to take which 'might or might not help, depending on the circumstances'. He then said that one of the nurses would explain what was to happen in more detail, when Richard's mother was present.

Richard responded that it was 'alright by him'. On leaving the consulting room, Richard was given a Patient Information Sheet and a consent form specifically designed for the clinical trial in question. The Patient Information Sheet clearly indicated that a placebo could be given and that side effects could occur during the administration of the treatment programme. Richard put the sheet in his pocket.

When Mrs Douglas reappeared, Richard told her that the doctor wanted him to try a new treatment. Mrs Douglas asked one of the nurses to explain, and was told that Richard would continue to receive the effective treatment, but would be involved in testing out a new drug which could enhance the standard treatment. Richard and his mother then both signed the consent form.

After two months of treatment with the inhaler and with a tablet the nature of which was unknown to Mrs Douglas and Richard, his asthma was stable, but his mother noticed a marked tendency to irritability in him, which she has not observed before. Concerned that this might be the result of the medication, she contacted the hospital and informed that consultant's secretary that she was not allowing Richard to take any more of the tablets.

From the review of the legal and non-legal controls over research in sections 10.2 and 10.3, it can be seen that Richard's case raises a number of areas for discussion. The issue of consent is particularly important in view of Richard's age, bearing in mind the possibility of legal action if that consent were not obtained in accordance with what would be regarded as proper practice. Similarly, legal and ethical difficulties are posed by the use of a randomized trial, and the influence of the Ethics Committee is relevant here. These, therefore, are the key issues which require further examination in the light of Richard's case.

10.5 Consent

General principles regarding consent are the subject of Chapter 6 – it is the legal issue of consent in relation to research which is addressed here.

10.5.1 *Consent in research projects*

In a situation such as Richard's, where patient care is combined with a research trial, it is important that the patient appreciates this dual role on the part of his carers. Unless the research is, for example, of a purely observational nature, then the subject must be aware of the fact that he is involved in a project [19]. This seems to be the case for Richard, but a factor which may not have been addressed by the consultant is that Richard may have felt some pressure to participate in the trial in order to oblige and seem willing to help. For consent to be truly voluntary it should be stressed to the patient that he or she is quite free to refuse to participate without any adverse response or sanction occurring and that the patient can also withdraw during the course of the trial if he wants to.

The way in which consent is obtained from the patient can also confirm or cast doubt on its validity. The UKCC advisory document, *Exercising Accountability* [20], warns that in respect of patients in hospital, there are good reasons why the information should be given and the consent sought in the presence of a nurse, and this may apply equally well to out-patient procedures. The Royal College of Physicians' Report [21] recommends a sliding scale of ways of obtaining consent. For example research involving less than minimal risk could proceed on the basis of oral consent given after an oral explanation. This would not be appropriate in Richard's case. His age, condition, and the fact that a reaction to the new form of treatment could be more than trivial indicates the need for written consent. This will then provide the necessary proof of consent in case of litigation and means that Richard is in no doubt that he is involved in something more than ordinary straightforward treatment. However the standard consent to treatment form is not regarded as acceptable by the Royal College of Physicians and it is therefore wise for any research team to devise a tailor-made form of consent for approval by the relevant Ethics Committee for use in the trial, rather than relying on the standard form.

In support of the consent form, the College recommends the use of a patient information sheet, which explains the investigation, and particularly the risks involved. In Richard's case, the consultant did not give any oral explanation of the reasons for the study, or the possible side effects which could result from the new therapy. Possibly the consultant may have expected this to be done by the nurse in the presence of Richard's mother, but this was not, in the event, the case. It was therefore left to Richard to glean the information from the sheet, yet he had little time to do so, and his mother was not aware of the existence of the sheet, due to Richard putting it into his pocket. Had the nurse to whom Richard and his mother spoke, realized from their questions that they had not understood the procedure, its risks and implications, then as the UKCC *Exercising Accountability* [22] document makes plain, it would be the responsibility of that nurse to arrange for them to speak to the consultant again so that the deficiencies could be remedied.

This is therefore a case, not uncommon in reality, where a sequence of coincidences means that best practice has not been followed. Standard practice requires a full explanation of the reasons for and risks of treatment: if this has not been forthcoming, then questions may be raised about the genuineness of Richard's consent and the duty of care of the health care team. In an ideal world, more time should have been given to Richard and his mother to reach a decision, and more information given either by the consultant or other members of the team as to the risks and benefits to Richard himself. In the circumstances given, it might be difficult to demonstrate that he had been adequately informed of the nature and general purpose of the study, and of the consequences for his own treatment.

The extent to which Richard really understood what was being proposed depends not only on the information he was given, but also on his capacity to comprehend the explanations offered. Special considerations arise when research is to be undertaken in patients who may have limited comprehension, and these issues will now be considered.

10.5.2 *Consent in special cases – children*

Department of Health guidelines for local research ethics committees draw a distinction between therapeutic and non-therapeutic research involving children [23]. The guidelines provide that 'research proposals should only involve children where it is absolutely essential to do so and the information required cannot be obtained using adult subjects'. Moreover if the proposal is for non-therapeutic research, then the child must be subject to no more than 'minimal risk'. It is thus acknowledged that research which adds to the biological and psychological knowledge of children can only be carried out on children, and is therefore necessary for progress in treatment and care. But it is also acknowledged that non-therapeutic research requires stronger justification.

This distinction between therapeutic and non-therapeutic research persists in the area of capacity to consent, with the added complication that the law relating to capacity of minors (children under the age of 18) to consent to medical treatment is far from straightforward. In most areas of the law minors are the subject of special provisions. The rules relating to the ability of a person under the age of 18 to permit medical treatment to be carried out reflect this need for different rules, with the additional complexity that a further distinction is drawn between minors generally and minors over the age of 16.

Where children over the age of 16 are concerned, the Family Law Reform Act 1969 states that a minor who has reached the age of 16 years is competent to give consent to medical treatment. This consent will be as valid as if the minor were of full age, and therefore consent of the parent or guardian is, by statute, unnecessary. The statute is concerned specifically with medical treatment however. Therefore whilst this rule would appear to give the necessary legal protection to medical researchers in a therapeutic setting, the Act does not apply to non-therapeutic research.

Where a minor is under the age of 16, the House of Lords decision in the celebrated case of *Gillick* v. *West Norfolk and Wisbech Area Health Authority* (1985) would appear to apply to therapeutic research. Thus if a child is 'Gillick-competent', i.e. has sufficient maturity and intelligence to understand the nature and implications of the proposed treatment, then parental consent is once again unnecessary and the child's agreement is regarded as effective in law. The age at which the necessary degree of understanding and maturity is reached will obviously vary from child to child.

In all other cases not covered by these rules, researchers will look to the parent or guardian of the child to provide the necessary consent. In the case of therapeutic research where the child may gain some benefit from the procedure, this proxy consent will be effective if it is in the best interests of the child. The child's wishes should never be ignored however. The Declaration of Helsinki states that even where the law allows parental consent to replace that of the patient, wherever the minor can give consent then that should be obtained in addition to that of the legal guardian. This point is developed in the Department of Health guidelines mentioned earlier which make it clear that the giving of consent by a parent or guardian cannot override the refusal of consent by a child who is competent to make that decision.

It is non-therapeutic research which poses the greatest difficulty where the question of consent is concerned. As noted before, the Family Law Reform Act 1969 has no application in these circumstances, and there is no authority on the question of whether or not the *Gillick* decision applies to non-therapeutic research. In theory, the *Gillick* case gave a general ruling concerning the ability of older children to make their own decisions, and therefore there is no reason why the general *Gillick* principle should not apply. In practice, the prudent researcher should seek parental consent in addition to that of a child of whatever age. But even here there is some uncertainty as to the precise effect of this process. It is in the duty of the parent to act in the best interests of the child. Strictly interpreted this could mean that a parent may only legally give consent to the child's participation in a trial if this would be for the benefit of the child. This creates obvious problems where non-therapeutic research carries no prospect of direct benefit, and may even present some risk for the child.

It is possible to construct an argument which justifies parental consent in these circumstances, based on a wider interpretation of the parent's duty [24]. Thus the parent's obligation could be seen as not to do anything which would be clearly against the interests of the child. If the risks involved in the study were minimal and the child would be rendering a service to the community, then the parent may be acting legally in agreeing to the procedure. The law is far from conclusive on this point however, and in the absence of any case law on the subject, there is a pressing need for statutory regulation. Researchers need to know who can validly give consent in these circumstances, and so for their protection, and the protection of young patients who are research subjects, legislation is needed to clarify the position.

So far as Richard Douglas is concerned, as he is under the age of 16 and is already a patient of the consultant, this would appear to be a case where the *Gillick* principle could be invoked. Certainly as regards standard practice, if it appeared to the consultant that Richard had the ability to understand the nature and implications of the proposed treatment, then he would be regarded as '*Gillick*-competent' and of sufficient capacity to consent to treatment. If, by analogy, the *Gillick* case can be applied to research, then Richard's consent could be valid. The obtaining of his mother's consent is a wise precaution, although the efficacy of her consent in this case has to be called into question as she was not aware of all the relevant facts at the time when she gave her agreement to the trial. In fact, in comparison with many parents who have misgivings about entering their children in trials, she seems a little over eager.

If Richard were not deemed sufficiently competent to give his own consent, however, problems could ensue. Jane Douglas's consent might be effective if it were in Richard's best interests – but it would not have been possible for her to assess this adequately in the circumstances. Richard's case highlights the need for clarification of the question of consent to research in children and also the procedures for gaining consent. It is here that the nursing members of the health care team can play a significant role in ensuring that consent is truly informed, in that both patient and parents fully understand the nature of the treatment, its risks and benefits.

10.5.3 *Consent in special cases – mental impairment*

In passing it is worth noting that the question of competence and capacity can be equally problematical when raised in the context of mentally impaired patients although this is considered more extensively in general terms in Chapter 8. The parameters of the argument in relation to research are set out clearly in World Health Organisation guidelines [25]:

> 'substantially similar ethical considerations apply to the mentally ill and the mentally handicapped as to children. They should never be the subjects of research that might equally well be carried out in adults in full possession of their intellectual faculties, but they are clearly the only subjects available for research into the origins and treatment of mental disease or disability.'

Many people who are mentally ill or mentally handicapped are in fact able to give valid consent to medical treatment, and, by analogy, to participation in research projects. Where that competence is not present however, there is no provision in law for another person to give consent by proxy to any research activity.

Regrettably, this is another situation where there is much ethical debate on the subject, but the all important legal regulation is lacking. In *F v. West Berkshire Health Authority* (1989), the House of Lords, considering the question of treatment of a person with mental handicap, ruled that in the absence of that person's ability to consent, it is still lawful to give general medical and surgical treatment and care provided it is in the best interests of the patient and in accordance with a responsible body of relevant professional opinion. A similar test may well be applicable to therapeutic research, but there is no legal sanction for this. And certainly there is, as yet, no indication as to how the law would regard non-therapeutic research involving the mentally impaired. However cogent the ethical arguments in favour of such activity, researchers are on dangerous ground at present.

10.6 Randomized controlled therapeutic trials

A further consideration in the case of Richard Douglas concerns the fact that the research programme in which he has been enlisted is based on a randomized controlled trial. Such trials are becoming increasingly common because of their usefulness as a research tool. Their most appropriate application is in cases where it is necessary to determine the efficacy of a new drug. By comparing the experience of one group of patients who receive the new drug (the treatment group) with a similar group who receive either no treatment or a different (probably the standard) treatment (the control group) it is possible to draw significant conclusions concerning the safety and effects of a new form of treatment.

As with the case of Richard Douglas members of the control group may receive an inert treatment – a placebo – instead of the drug under consideration. To eliminate the danger of subjectivity, the trial may be conducted under 'double blind' conditions, where the investigator who assesses the patients is not aware of which treatment those patients are receiving, and the patients are allocated at random to the treatment group or control group.

Such randomized trials contain a number of in-built ethical and moral problems. A new treatment which may have adverse side effects is being used on one group of patients but, at the same time, if that treatment proves to be a genuine improvement on the standard therapy, then an effective treatment is being denied to the control group. Moreover, such trials create a conflict of obligations for the physician concerned, between the duty to patients and the furtherance of medical knowledge.

From a legal point of view, there is again no specific case law or legislation which governs the use of such trials, or provides guidance to a researcher as to their legality or otherwise. All that can be said at present is that the obtaining of fully informed consent seems to be the key factor in determining whether a particular randomized controlled trial is truly within legal limits. This is itself creates problems, as the patient cannot be told which treatment they will receive. But to enter a patient in such a trial without some explanation, and some indication of consent to this, renders the researcher liable to an action for battery. There must therefore be a proper explanation to the patient, in terms that can be understood, of the random nature of the trial. Provided Richard Douglas has given his consent freely in full understanding of what is involved, then as the law stands at present those caring for him will have done everything they can to ensure that they remain within the law.

10.7 Review of research and compensation

Once a research project has been approved by an Ethics Committee and is under way, the conduct of that research is wholly in the hands of the health care team. There is no formal provision for review of the project by an Ethics Committee or any other independent person or body. It has been suggested [26] that some mechanism should exist whereby Ethics Committees can influence research more fully, for example by requiring investigators to produce a brief report of progress, at least annually – but at present no such arrangements exist. The subjects of research depend for protection wholly on the investigators' sense of professional duty towards them. No legal controls or sanctions are invoked unless and until a project goes so badly wrong that the need to establish liability and the right to compensation arises.

Where a patient has been harmed by some invasive procedure or by exposure to drugs during the course of the trial, the right to compensation will depend on proof of negligence on the part of the research investigator, one or more members of the team or the supplier of the drug, or on proof that a 'producer' has supplied a 'defective' product under the Consumer Protection Act 1987. The cost of pursuing an action in negligence, in economic and in human terms, mean that this is not a course of action to be undertaken lightly. Nor is the Consumer Protection Act 1987 necessarily the answer to the problem, as the manufacturer may be able to argue that a side effect or outcome could not have been discovered in the light of current scientific and technical knowledge and that a 'state of the art' defence is therefore available.

Litigation on either of these grounds can be lengthy, expensive, and its outcome uncertain, and many different bodies, from the Medical Research Council to Action for Victims of Medical Accidents, recognize that compensation for subjects injured during the course of research should be placed on a more satisfactory basis. Ex gratia schemes exist whereby the Department of Health and the Association of the British Pharmaceutical Industry (ABPI) will pay compensation without admitting liability, but this is in the nature of a discretionary payment rather than a right. Moreover the ABPI scheme draws a distinction between healthy volunteers and patients, treating healthy volunteers on a more favourable basis – an invidious distinction as a patient who agrees to subject himself to risk surely deserves better [27].

Returning to the case study, if Mrs Douglas is thinking of claiming compensation for the apparent change in Richard's health, then the prospects are not good. An initial difficulty is the issue of causation, for it will have to be shown that the change in Richard's behaviour is in fact due to the tablets he has taken. If of course he has been given the placebo, the case could not proceed on the ground of adverse reaction to a drug. But if he has been given the experimental drug, then negligence or liability under the Consumer Protection Act 1987 will have to be proved before any legal redress is available.

In the event, Mrs Douglas removes him from the trial, and assuming Richard himself agrees to this, this must be accepted by the research team, and no further participation must be expected of Richard, nor must any adverse consequences follow in respect of his treatment.

10.8 Conclusions

The above overview of the law and its application to the case study should give some indication of the difficulties which surround research involving patients. One of the chief difficulties is the lack of clear, legally enforceable rules in two crucial areas. One area is that of consent, where researchers are at the mercy of rather vague guidelines. The other area concerns the absence of legal control over the conduct of research and the absence of adequate provision for compensation if that research leads to injury.

Considerable discussion and reform of the law is required to ensure that researchers and patients can rely on clear guidelines as to their responsibilities and rights, and that the necessary legal safeguards are in place to protect those patients who agree to serve the community through participation in medical research.

10.9 Notes and references

1. See the definition given in Royal College of Physicians, *Research Involving Patients*, London: Royal College of Physicians, 1990.
2. Royal College of Physicians, *Guidelines on the Practice of Ethics Committees in Medical Research involving Human Subjects*, 2nd edn., London: Royal College of Physicians, 1990.
3. Royal College of Physicians, *Guidelines on the Practice of Ethics Committees in Medical Research involving Human Subjects*, 2nd edn., London: Royal College of Physicians, 1990.
4. Mason, J.K., McCall Smith, *Law and Medical Ethics*, 4th edn., London: Butterworths, 1994.
5. The distinction between therapeutic and non-therapeutic research was drawn by the Declaration of Helsinki produced by the World Medical Association in 1964. This declaration provides the foundation values for the conduct of all biomedical research.
6. The Declaration of Helsinki (revised 1989).

7. Nicholson, R.H., ed. *Medical Research with Children*. p 26.

8. See references 1 and 2.

9. UKCC, *The Code of Professional Conduct for the Nurse, Midwife and Health Visitor*, 3rd edn., London: UKCC, 1992.

10. Kennedy, I., Grubb, A., *Medical Law: Texts and Materials*, 1st edn., London: Butterworths, 1989.

11. UKCC, *Exercising Accountability*, London: UKCC, 1989.

12. The Nuremberg Code 1949.

13. For the full text of the Declaration of Helsinki, see Kennedy, I., Grubb, A., *Medical Law: Texts and Materials*, 1st edn., London: Butterworths, 1989: p 865.

14. (i) Royal College of Physicians, *Research Involving Patients*, London: Royal College of Physicians, 1990.
    (ii) Royal College of Physicians, *Guidelines on the Practice of Ethics Committees in Medical Research involving Human Subjects*, 2nd edn., London: Royal College of Physicians, 1990.
    (iii) Royal College of Physicians, *Research on Healthy Volunteers*, London: Royal College of Physicians, 1986.

15. RCN, *Ethics related to Research in Nursing*, Harrow: Scutari Press, 1993.

16. Royal College of Physicians, *Guidelines on the Practice of Ethics Committees in Medical Research involving Human Subjects*, 2nd edn., London: Royal College of Physicians, 1990: p 3.

17. Faulder, C., *Whose Body is it Anyway?*, London, Virago Press, 1985.

18. British Medical Association, *Handbook of Medical Ethics*, London: BMA, 1988.

19. British Medical Association, *Handbook of Medical Ethics*, London: BMA, 1988.

20. UKCC, *Exercising Accountability*, London: UKCC, 1989.

21. Royal College of Physicians, *Research Involving Patients*, London: Royal College of Physicians, 1990.

22. UKCC, *Exercising Accountability*, London: UKCC, 1989.

23. Department of Health, *Local Research Ethics Committees* HSG(91)5, London: , 1991.

24. See Brazier, M., *Medicine, Patients and the Law*, 2nd edn., Harmondsworth, Penguin, 1992: pp 421–3.

25. World Health Organisation, *Proposed international guidelines for biomedical research involving human subjects*, Geneva: WHO, 1982.

26. Royal College of Physicians, *Research Involving Patients*, London: Royal College of Physicians, 1990.

27. See Brazier, M., *Medicine Patients and the Law*, 2nd edn., Harmondsworth, Penguin, 1992.

B An Ethical Perspective – Nursing Research
Alison Dines

10.10 Introduction

Nurses may be interested in the ethical issues raised by research with patients and clients from two contrasting standpoints. Firstly from the perspective of a practitioner working with patients who may be involved in research as subjects. Secondly from the viewpoint of a researcher who may be asking clients to participate in a particular project. This section of the chapter will explore both these elements. It will become apparent that there are important ethical principles that unite the two perspectives.

The Code of Professional Conduct for the Nurse, Midwife and Health Visitor [1] provides standards by which all registered nurses are expected to practise and conduct themselves. Much of this framework is of immediate relevance to the practitioner or researcher when considering ethical issues in research. More recently the research advisory group of one professional organization, the Royal College of Nursing (RCN), has produced the document *Ethics Related to Nursing Research* [2] . This explores the responsibilities of

- nurses undertaking research
- nurses practising in settings where research is being undertaken and
- nurses in positions of authority where research is to be carried out.

Both of these documents will be utilized in the following discussion.

The theme of the discussion is the tension between protecting a patient's interests and conducting research. In the first part informed consent is proposed as – in general – the most adequate way to reconcile this tension. The latter part of the chapter explores this patient interest/research theme through a particular example of nursing research.

10.11 The Code of Conduct – the inherent dilemma

The Code of Conduct states that,

'each registered nurse, midwife and health visitor shall act, at all times, in such a manner as to:

- safeguard and promote the interests of individual patients and clients;
- serve the interests of society;

- justify public trust and confidence and
- uphold and enhance the good standing ... of the professions.'

This provides a useful starting point for considering the ethical issues related to research with patients.

An examination of these first two phrases that nurses should 'safeguard and promote the interests of individual patients and clients' and 'serve the interests of society' embodies a tension that is at the heart of any research with patients. Research by its very nature, as has been discussed earlier in the chapter, is primarily concerned to advance knowledge which it is hoped may serve the interests of society, including benefitting future patients. The nurse by conducting research herself or by facilitating research with patients with whom she works thereby responds to this requirement of the Code of Conduct. The research process, however, may or may not benefit the individual patient presently participating in the research, yet the Code of Conduct also requires that the nurse should safeguard and promote the interests of individual patients and clients in her work. How this safeguarding and protecting is to be done in practice raises some difficult questions for the nurse which are made more complex by her dual loyalty to society as well as the patient.

10.11.1 *Promoting benefit and minimizing harm*

If the nurse is to 'safeguard and promote the interests of individual patients and clients', how might this influence any research she undertakes or her view of any requests for research with patients with whom she is practising? The nurse may interpret the need to promote the interests of patients as a primary concern that patients will *benefit* from any research in which they participate. According to this view therapeutic research with its attempt to benefit patients on whom it is carried out might be deemed acceptable. In contrast non-therapeutic research where patients are unlikely to be benefitted by the procedure will be rejected. The type of research in which Richard Douglas (in the case study) was invited to participate was therapeutic research and would be deemed ethically acceptable according to this standard.

The nurse may alternatively interpret the need to safeguard the interests of clients as a responsibility to minimize the harm to which patients are exposed. In this case non-therapeutic research will again be rejected both by nurse-researchers and practitioners as it inevitably exposes patients to harm. This is because in a minimal sense any research will involve some 'interference' with a patient's life, more generally it may also involve other harms such as invasion of privacy or exposure to certain risks and hazards. Therapeutic research might also be rejected on the grounds of minimizing exposure to harms. For example, patients are invited to take part in a randomized controlled trial which compares a traditional treatment with a low potential for harm but also low potential benefit, with a new treatment where there is a potential for high benefit but also high risk of harm. If the nurse is primarily concerned to minimize the harm to which patients are exposed then the traditional treatment will be preferred with its avoidance of greater potential harm and the request for the patient to participate in such research will be resisted. In a similar vein a nurse-researcher may decide any experimental studies that she might be contemplating, though yielding valuable findings are ethically unacceptable. In the case study it is possible that the double blind randomized controlled trial in which Richard Douglas was asked to participate would also be viewed as ethically unacceptable according to this 'preventing harm' view.

The wholesale rejection of non-therapeutic research for patients, and possibly some therapeutic research, effectively prevents the further development of many advances in health care. This is a price which to some might seem excessive and even unethical in view of the potential benefits to future patients and clients.

10.11.2 *Research for the good of society*

If the nurse is to 'serve the interests of society' how might this influence her research work or her view of any requests for research with patients with whom she is practising? If the nurse adopts this as her primary standard against which requests for research with patients are measured and any nursing research studies are designed, then both therapeutic and non-therapeutic research will be deemed acceptable. Both are likely to either benefit patients or generate new knowledge thereby serving the interests of society. It might also be possible that using this measure the nurse conducts and accepts research that does *not* safeguard and promote the *individual* interests of patients and clients. Thus, to take an extreme example, research designed to follow the natural course of breast cancer in women might require that a large number of women are left untreated and the progress of their disease monitored. This research may be of tremendous benefit to society as the natural history of breast cancer is poorly understood, the interests of the individual patients and clients, however, would be totally overridden in this quest for new knowledge. If the nurse judged research *only* on the basis of the interest of society such research would be deemed acceptable.

10.12 Paternalism, utilitarianism and respect for persons

None of the above responses offer an approach to research with patients that is intuitively acceptable. The emphasis purely upon the patient's individual interests seems to demand the rejection of many forms of research. The alternative emphasis primarily upon the interest of society seems to accept abuse of patients and clients for the greater good of society. A different ethical basis for research with patients and clients is called for. The discussion above demonstrates ethical approaches based upon **paternalism** in the first case and **utilitarianism** in the second. In a paternalistic approach judgments are made on behalf of patients by the care-giver, in this case the nurse. In utilitarianism the greatest good for society is the sole criterion, with the unpalatable consequence that individuals may be 'used' for the greater benefit of society.

An approach that potentially enables the nurse to both safeguard and promote the interests of individuals whilst at the same time serve the interests of society, is one where **respect for persons** is the paramount criterion. The main way in which such respect is demonstrated when undertaking research is through **informed consent**. Of course informed consent can only apply where the individual concerned is competent to be involved in decision-making. Where this does not apply then the decision, once more, will entail a balancing of paternalism and utilitarianism. The 'consent' of a surrogate can be sought, but there may be a presumption that (with the exception of low risk therapeutic research) research should not be conducted without the informed consent of the individuals concerned.

10.12.1 *Informed consent*

Informed consent does appear to overcome some of the difficulties outlined above. Thus if an individual patient has sufficient information to judge the merits of a particular research project then, even if it is non-therapeutic and will not directly benefit them personally, they may choose to be involved as they wish to help future patients. Similarly if therapeutic research exposes a person to a greater potential for harm then the individual may choose to take this risk knowing that the potential for benefit is also increased. The patients – through informed consent – are recognized to be in the best position to judge their own interests which may at times be to practice altruism or to take known risks.

Informed consent will also prevent abuse of patients out of a concern to benefit society. Thus if patients or clients are fully informed about both therapeutic and non-therapeutic research including those that pose considerable hazards to them personally, then the likelihood of over-riding individual interests is considerably reduced. The wording of the Code of Conduct that 'each registered nurse . . . shall . . . safeguard and promote the interests of individual patients and clients' allows for informed consent to non-therapeutic research or increased risks of harm as it does not identify *who* is to be the judge of the patient's interests. The advantages of informed consent outlined above might also contribute to meeting the requirement that nurses 'justify public trust and confidence and uphold and enhance the good standing ... of the professions' through the avoidance of abuse in research and by playing a part in the development of research-based practice.

10.12.2 *Lay and professional views of information*

It was mentioned earlier in section 10.4.1 that the Nuremberg Code of 1949 indicates that the voluntary consent of the human subject is absolutely essential. Veatch [3] suggests that consent giving can be seen as the negotiation of a contract. Consent, he writes, requires that, 'all potentially useful or meaningful information be transmitted.' An important question that is raised by this concerns who is to decide what is potentially useful or meaningful information? The section 10.2.1 discussed how legally this is usually taken to be a professional decision i.e. what a reasonable doctor (or nurse) would have disclosed under the circumstances.

This poses a number of problems however. The first concerns the fact that 'there are enormous differences between doctors in the amount of information they see fit to give their patients' [4]. Relying upon a professional standard also assumes that professionals are in the best position to make such judgments. Decisions about what patients might wish to know about research projects include not only technical issues but those based upon personal values and beliefs; the researcher might value very different information about the research than the patient. It is in recognition of these limitations that there is now a movement for greater lay involvement in decisions about what patients might wish to know when being asked to participate in research. In parallel with this is a consumer movement which aims to educate members of the public about what questions *to ask* when invited to take part in research.

There are of course different difficulties which emerge when professional judgments about 'what patients would wish to know' are replaced by lay evaluations. The lay representatives cannot represent the full spectrum of human variation. Thus one person may wish to have an unusually high level of knowledge about a research project and another may express a desire not to know anything. Judgments made on the basis of what patients *generally* might wish to know would not cater for these differing needs. One practical way of overcoming these differing desires for information is, as Veatch, suggests, to ask people what they wish to know! He writes, 'the researcher's job will be to create a climate where the subject can express uniqueness in this way.'

10.12.3 *What information is to be conveyed?*

The Patient's Charter [5] reaffirms the right that patients have to 'be given a clear explanation of any treatment proposed, including any risks and any alternatives, before you decide whether you will agree to treatment'. It also acknowledges the right to 'choose whether or not you wish to take part in medical research'. Both these statements are in keeping with the need for informed consent to research.

Various attempts have been made to outline in practical terms the type of information to which patients should have access if they are to give or refuse their informed consent to research. The RCN [6] sees this as requiring that the

> 'researcher explain as fully as possible, and in terms meaningful to the subjects, the nature and purpose of the study, how and why they were selected and invited to take part, what is required of them and who is undertaking and financing the investigation.'

In addition emphasis is given to the subject's absolute right to refuse to participate or to withdraw from the study without their care being affected in any way.

Veatch [7] has more specifically identified some key information that he feels must be imparted. This includes:

- acknowledgement if the design of the research includes a control group,
- information about any 'inconveniences' of the research as well as risks and discomforts,
- a named person for subjects to contact for further information about the research,
- the right of patients to alternative treatment to that proposed in the research project,
- identification of who is responsible for any harms that may accrue from the research and
- acknowledgement of the right to continue any helpful treatment.

Two organizations have addressed these issues directly from the patient's perspective, reviewing the questions that patients might wish to ask themselves and others if they are to participate in research. Eagle in the Channel 4 television *Today's health service – a user's guide* [8] provides a checklist of questions for patients to ask if they are invited to take part in clinical trials. These include, for example,

- What will happen to the results of the research?
- What can be done to make me better if I get a problem while taking part?

- Can I have time to think about whether to take part?
- Would I get compensation if it all goes wrong for me?

A similar user-centred purpose lies behind a leaflet, *Medical research and you* [9] produced by an organization called CERES, (Consumers for Ethics in Research) which aims to promote informed debate about research and to involve users in every stage of health research. Written in an accessible style the leaflet looks at some of the questions that people may wish to ask such as

- What will happen to me?
- What will happen if I say 'no'?
- Do I have to decide at once?
- Is there written information I can keep about the research – to read when I'm thinking whether to take part – or to talk over with my friends?

The CERES leaflet also explains in simple terms about randomized trials, blind trials and placebos. In addition it prompts the patient or client to ask themselves, when thinking about such trials, do I mind being put into any group or do I want to choose my treatment, and would I mind being in a group having 'dummy treatment' (a placebo)?

A useful guide for nurse-researchers who may be involved in writing information for patients and clients being asked to take part in research is provided by CERES. The document, '*Spreading the word on research or patient information: how can we get it better*? provides practical ideas about such work [10]. It recommends, for example, using short words, sentences and paragraphs, using requests rather than commands, writing in the active voice (we will book) rather than the passive (appointments will be booked) and taking a personal approach (we, you, your baby) rather than the impersonal (they, those, he or she).

10.12.4 *Patients as partners in research*

The existence of the attempts by Channel 4 and CERES to empower health care users with meaningful questions when faced with research is evidence of an increasing shift in health care from a paternalistic focus to one of working increasingly in partnership with patients. This is an approach that has been welcomed, at least in theory if not in practice, by the profession of nursing and receives an ethical grounding in 'respect for persons' [11]. Veatch entitles his book, *The patient as partner* and in keeping with much current thinking he rejects an approach to research that treats patients as passive subject 'material'. In contrast he calls for a recognition of the lay decision-maker as a questioning, thinking, feeling, active moral person.

10.13 Justice and promise keeping

Veatch suggests that in addition to considerations of doing good, avoiding harm and respect for persons, those concerned with ethical issues related to research with patients should also be concerned with the principles of justice and the need to respect a patient's privacy and maintain confidentiality. These will now be briefly considered.

10.13.1 The choice of participants

The question of justice in research focuses upon, for example, the issue of how participants are selected to take part in the research. Two plausible interpretations of justice see this as either a concern to maximize the position of the least well-off members of a society or an attempt to get the distribution of benefits and burdens as equal as possible. The implications of these views for conducting research are that any patient, as by definition a less 'well-off' member of society, who is asked to participate in research must on balance be expected to benefit from participating. If this is not expected to be the case, then it may be unjust or unfair to ask the patient or client to participate in the first place. This may pose problems for researchers as it can be argued that frequently research does *not* provide a net benefit to participants when, for example, the inconvenience of involvement and the risk of unanticipated side effects is remembered. Veatch suggests it may then only be possible to accept research as being just if the benefits to participants are combined with the benefits to society, provided of course that there is informed consent. If it is possible to carry out the research without burdening already 'disadvantaged' patients then this should be attempted. This is often not possible in health care research as the subject of interest is the patient or client with that particular health problem. This does raise some important questions about 'over researching' groups such as cancer patients or people with AIDS. The RCN guidance recognizes this concern with justice in selecting research subjects and suggests not imposing on them unnecessarily.

10.13.2 Privacy

Privacy concerns the right to keep or remove information from public knowledge and observation. It is closely related to matters of confidentiality which Sissela Bok suggests, 'refer to the boundaries surrounding shared secrets and to the process of guarding these boundaries' [12]. The Code of Conduct requires nurses to

> 'protect all confidential information concerning patients and clients obtained in the course of professional practice and make disclosures

only with consent, where required by the order of a court or where you can justify disclosure in the wider public interest.'

The RCN, in its advisory document, suggests [13] in the context of research that

'usually this means that data are analysed and reported in such a way that particular individuals, small groups, or even organisations cannot be identified unless they have given prior agreement, the full information being known only to the research team.'

10.14 Ethical review of the Richard Douglas case study

An important issue when considering the case of Richard Douglas is the adequacy of the consent given by Richard and his mother from an ethical viewpoint. The RCN suggest that the

'researcher explain as fully as possible, and in terms meaningful to the subjects, the nature and purpose of the study, how and why they were selected and invited to take part, what is required of them and who is undertaking and financing the investigation.'

According to these criteria the encounter by Mrs Douglas and Richard with both the consultant and the nurse fails to meet this ethical standard as a very full explanation was not given, no explicit mention of why Richard had been selected was made and the issue of financing was left undiscussed.

The suggestion that Richard would be 'really helpful' if he joined the study may be criticized as exercising some degree of coercion over him. The Nuremberg Code speaks of *voluntary* consent. Richard is in a vulnerable position as a patient and as a minor. It might be acceptable to encourage a person to participate in health care research if at the same time it is made clear that participation is entirely the person's free choice and he or she is free to refuse without jeopardizing any health care treatment.

A second difficulty with the discussion between Richard and the consultant and Mrs Douglas, Richard and the nurse, is that no verbal mention is made of any harms that might accrue from participation, nor that this is a randomized controlled trial. The written material does contain such detail but it can be argued that such information sheets should not be a substitute for a full discussion, rather a supplement and reinforcer for the person to consider at their leisure.

Further criticisms concern the absence of Richard's mother for much of the conversation with the consultant. As has been mentioned in section 10.5.2 although Richard is able to give his consent on the basis of being 'Gillick-competent' it is a 'wise precaution' to obtain the consent of his mother. The consultant therefore had an ethical duty to ensure Mrs Douglas too was party to the information about the project. The fact that Mrs Douglas may only discover the patient information sheet in Richard's pocket when the family washing is next done bears witness to the inadequacy of the way the encounter was handled from an ethical viewpoint! It is interesting to postulate that Mrs Douglas' and Richard's withdrawal from the research at a later date may possibly have been averted if the request to participate had been handled in a more 'person respecting' manner.

An improved approach on behalf of the consultant and the nurse would have been to ask for Richard's participation on one visit to the hospital, discussing the implications in full and supplying an information sheet to take away. Their consent could have been sought on the next visit after they had time to reflect.

10.15 The nurse-researcher dilemma

The tension between the need to 'safeguard and promote the interests of individual patients and clients' and 'serve the interests of society' in general medical research was mentioned in section 10.11. A similarly difficult issue lies at the heart of nursing research. A nurse in her practice might loosely be said to be concerned to offer direct benefit to patients in her care. A researcher offers the possibility of future benefit to patients by increasing understanding of nursing care. This different emphasis creates dilemmas in practice that will now be considered.

10.15.1 *Nurse-researcher case study*

A nurse-researcher is interested in the feeding problems of stroke patients. She is using non-participant observation as her research method. She is seated inconspicuously wearing a white coat in the ward, it is a meal time. A stroke patient nearby is propped up against his pillows and reaches for his milky tea. He takes the spouted beaker to his lips but spills the drink down his pyjama jacket. No nurse is in sight, what should the nurse-researcher do?

Some time later, the sister appears, she is updating the fluid balance charts. Observing the empty beaker she congratulates the patient on drinking his tea and charts the fluid intake. What should the nurse researcher do?

10.15.2 *Practical points*

The nurse-researcher in this scenario might feel a dual loyalty both to the patient and to her research. An immediate response might be to assist the patient when he spills his drink or at least to call a nurse on duty for help. Similarly when the sister incorrectly charts the patient's fluid balance the nurse-researcher might feel compelled to intervene and tell the sister what actually happened. All these responses would be in keeping with the Code of Professional Conduct with its guidance that nurses should, 'safeguard and promote the interests of individual patients and client.'

Alternatively the nurse-researcher might feel that to intervene in such a way might jeopardize the research. Thus assisting the patient with his drink or drying his front or even changing his jacket is contrary to the non-participant role the researcher is adopting. Any of these responses might contaminate the research findings as the nurse-researcher no longer discovers, for example, how long a patient might be left like this by everyday nursing practice or what action a ward nurse might take when discovering such a situation, both of which are pertinent to the feeding problems of stroke patients.

In addition if the nurse-researcher constantly intervenes every time she sees an occurrence like this then her presence in the ward environment may be resented by the ward nurses. They may begin to see her as a critical figure and may actually be on guard to ensure any practice within the nurse-researcher's sight is exemplary, once again distorting the research findings. All these reasons provide strong *practical* reasons for the nurse-researcher to refrain from intervening in such situations.

10.15.3 Ethical points

An important question is whether it is ethically acceptable for the nurse-researcher to do nothing in this situation in order to safeguard her research or is she ethically compelled to intervene even if it might jeopardize her research findings? The Code of Conduct provides one possible support for non-intervention when it says, 'ensure that no action or omission on your part, or *within your sphere of responsibility*, is detrimental to the interests, condition or safety of patients and clients.' It could be argued that the nurse-researcher, having agreed a non-participant status with the ward team, does not have any ethical responsibilities *as a nurse* to the patients on the ward. Support for this is provided by the RCN guideline,

> 'The nurse who is undertaking a research project in an exclusively research role has no responsibility for the service, care, treatment or advice given to patients or clients unless stipulated within the design of the research. Otherwise, any intervention in a professional capacity should be confined to situations in which a patient or client requires to be protected or rescued from danger [14].'

The degree of danger facing the patient in the scenario appears to be of crucial importance. It might be suggested that the spilling of milky tea does not pose a real danger. The milk is likely to have cooled the drink and, though the spillage may be humiliating for the patient, it does not pose a great physical danger of burning. The second situation in the scenario is more difficult to judge, one isolated occasion when a patient's fluid balance chart is incorrectly completed may not pose too great a threat. An accumulation of such incidents certainly would pose a threat as a patient is likely to become dehydrated.

Perhaps the decision about intervention is best left to the researcher's discretion in the particular situation she faces. Thus if over a period of hours this patient does not receive an adequate fluid intake there may be a moral imperative to intervene on the grounds of preventing patient harm even though this may jeopardize the research. The RCN Code is in line with this thinking.

'A nurse in a research situation still holds expert knowledge, and many at times feel impelled to action for a patient's benefit.'

Some additional ethical support for non-intervention is provided by the view that a nurse, or anyone, who undertakes research is bound to conduct the study to the highest standards in order both to enhance the validity of any findings and to help justify the intrusion into clients' and patients' lives. Non-intervention, by reducing contamination of the research findings, contributes to this imperative.

A non-intervention approach does demand, at the very least, a commitment to sharing the research findings directly with the ward staff concerned at the end of the study. Once again this corresponds to the requirement of the Code of Conduct that the nurse should, 'report to an appropriate person ... any circumstances that could jeopardise safe standards of practice'. Additionally, the nurse should assist 'professional colleagues ... to develop their professional competence'.

It has been suggested that the maxim 'behave as a responsible visitor' may provide a useful guide for these difficult situations. Thus a responsible visitor in the scenario might do something to help the patient if it appeared harm was likely to be caused by the spilled drink, alternatively in more difficult situations the responsible visitor might find a nurse to intervene if the problem was beyond a lay person's expertise. Occasionally a visitor might ignore a situation if the risk is not too great and it is felt important not to invade another person's private space in the ward. The difficulty of this analogy is that a nurse-researcher is unlike a visitor in that she *does* have expert knowledge and this may place some moral imperative upon her to use her knowledge for the patient's benefit. Certainly if there was a fire alarm then it would seem irresponsible for a nurse-researcher (and possibly even a visitor) not to assist in the evacuation of patients, and in the case of cardiac arrest she might diagnose the problem, sound the alarm and assist in resuscitation.

In these senses perhaps, as the RCN acknowledges, 'with specialist knowledge and skills it may be unacceptable to act just as a "good citizen".'

10.16 Conclusion

This ethical review of research with patients has identified two important issues both acknowledged by the RCN in its ethical guidelines for nurses. The first is the importance of 'an awareness that ethics in relation to current research in nursing cannot be considered outside the nursing context'. In other words, assessing research as a nurse involves reference both to the values of the profession and the practical demands of professional nursing practice. In addition assessment demands a recognition of the 'inherent potential conflict of perceived responsibilities for nurses who are involved in research in health care situations'. Awareness and debate among nurses about these issues is the first step to ensuring that our response to any research with patients is an ethical one.

10.17 Notes and references

Acknowledgement

I would like to thank Dr Elizabeth Carr, Visiting Research Fellow, Department of Nursing Studies, King's College, London, for the original idea for the nurse-researcher case study which is based upon an actual example encountered in her PhD research.

1. UKCC *Code of Professional Conduct for the Nurse, Midwife and Health Visitor*, London: UKCC, 1992.
2. RCN *Ethics Related to Research in Nursing*, Harrow: Scutari Press, 1993.
3. Veatch, R. *The patient as partner. A theory of human-experimentation ethics*, Bloomington: Indiana University Press, 1987: p 48.
4. Veatch, R. *The patient as partner. A theory of human-experimentation ethics*, Bloomington: Indiana University, Press, 1987: p 10.
5. Department of Health *The Patient's Charter*, London: HMSO, 1991.
6. RCN *Ethics Related to Research in Nursing*, Harrow: Scutari Press, 1993.
7. Veatch, R. The patient as partner. A theory of human-experimentation ethics, Bloomington: Indiana University Press, 1987.
8. Eagle, R. *Today's health service – a user's guide*, London: Broadcasting Support Services, Channel 4 Television, 1993.
9. CERES *Medical research and you*, London: CERES, 1993.
10. Alderson, P. *Spreading the word on research or patient information:*

how can we get it better? London: CERES, 1993. Postal application can be made for either of the CERES leaflets to: P O Box 1365, London, N16 0BW.

11. Meyer, J. 'Lay participation in care: threat to the status quo', in Wilson Barnett, J., Macleod Clark, J. *Research in health promotion and nursing.* London: Macmillan, 1993.

12. Bok, S. *Secrets: On the ethics of concealment and revelation*, Oxford: Oxford University Press, 1984.

13. RCN *Ethics Related to Research in Nursing*, Harrow: Scutari Press, 1993.

14. RCN *Ethics Related to Research in Nursing*, Harrow: Scutari Press, 1993.

Appendix
Further Reading

Beauchamp, T.L. and Childress, J.F. (1989) *Principles of Biomedical Ethics*, Oxford University Press, Oxford.

Benjamin, M. & Curtis, J. (1992) *Ethics in Nursing*, Oxford University Press, Oxford.

Brazier, M. (1992) *Medicine, Patients and the Law*, 2nd edn, Penguin Books, Meddlesex.

Chadwick, R. & Tadd, W. (1992), *Ethics and Nursing Practice: A Case Study Approach*, Macmillan, Basingstoke, Hampshire.

Dingwall, R. *et al.* (1991), *Medical Negligence: A Review and Bibliography*, Centre for Socio-Legal Studies, Oxford.

Dimond, B. (1990), *Legal Aspects of Nursing*, Prentice Hall, Hemel Hempstead, Herts.

Dimond, B. (1993) *Patient's Rights Responsibilities and the Nurse*, Central Health Studies Series, Quay Press, Lancaster.

Dyer, C. (1992) *Doctors, Patients and the Law*, Blackwell Scientific Publications, Oxford.

Gilligan, C. (1982) *In a Different Voice*, Harvard University Press, Cambridge, Mass.

Gillon, R. (1985) *Philosophical Medical Ethics*, John Wiley and Sons, Chichester.

Gillon, R. (1994) *Principles of Health Care Ethics*, John Wiley and Sons, Chichester.

Grubb, A. (Ed) (1992), *Challenges in Medical Care*, John Wiley and Sons, Chichester.

Hodgson, J. (1993) *Employment Law for Nurses*, Central Health Studies Series, Quay Press, Lancaster.

Holliday, I. (1992), *The NHS Transformed*, Baseline Books, Manchester.

Johnstone, M.J. (1989) *Bioethics – A Nursing Perspective*, Bailliere Tindall, London.

Jones, M.A. (1991) *Medical Negligence*, Sweet and Maxwell, London.

Kennedy, I. & Grubb, A. (1994) *Medical Law: Texts and Materials*, 2nd edn, Butterworths, London.

Longley, D. (1993), *Public Law and Health Service Accountability*, Open University Press, Buckingham.

Mason, J.K. & McCall Smith, A. (1994) *Law and Medical Ethics*, 4th edn, Butterworths, London.

Northrop, C.E. & Kelly, M.E. (1987) *Legal Issues in Nursing,* The C.V. Mosby Company, Washington.

Pyne, R.H. (1992), *Professional Discipline in Nursing, Midwifery and Health Visiting,* 2nd Ed, Blackwell Scientific Publications, Oxford.

RCN (1993) *Ethics Related to Research in Nursing,* Scutari Press, Harrow.

Rumbold, G. (1993) *Ethics in Nursing Practice,* Bailliere Tindall, London.

Seedhouse, D. (1988) *Ethics: The Heart of Health Care,* John Wiley and Sons, Chichester.

Singer, P. (ed) (1993) *A Companion to Ethics,* Blackwells, Oxford.

Thompson, I., Melia, K.M., Boyd, K.M. (1988) *Nursing Ethics,* Churchill Livingstone, Edinburgh.

UKCC (1989) *Exercising Accountability,* UKCC, London.

UKCC (1992) *Code of Professional Conduct for the Nurse, Midwife and Health Visitor,* UKCC, London.

Young, A.P. (1989) *Legal Problems in Nursing Practice,* 2nd Ed Chapman and Hall, London.

Young, A.P. (1991) *Law and Professional Conduct in Nursing,* Scutari Press, Harrow, Middx.

Young, A.P. (1992) *Case Studies in Law and Nursing: A Course Book for Project 2000 Training,* Chapman Hall, London.

Journals

Bulletin of Medical Ethics, Professional and Scientific Publications Ltd, London.

European Journal of Health Law, Kluwer Academic Publishers, The Netherlands.

Health Care Analysis, John Wiley & Sons, Chichester

Health Care Risk Report, The Eclipse Group, London.

Journal of Medical Ethics, BMJ Publishing Group for the Institute of Medical Ethics and the BMA.

Medical Law International, AB Academic Publishers, Bicester, Oxon.

Medical Law Review, published by Oxford University Press in Association with The Centre of Medical Law and Ethics, King's College, London.

Nursing Ethics, published by Edward Arnold, London.

Publications from Professional Healthcare Organisations

The doctors' medical defence organisations also provide some inexpensive well produced literature on medico-legal problems. Their publications are free to their medical, nursing and dental members. To non-members a small charge is made. Write to the organisations for their current publications list.

Publications Section
The Medical Defence Union
3 Devonshire Place
London Wl 2EA

Publications Section
The Medical Protection Society
50 Hallam Street
London
WIN 6DE.

AVMA (Action for Victims of Medical Accidents) also produce some useful medico-legal publications. Ask for their publications list.

AVMA
Bank Chambers
1 London Road
London
SE23 3TP

Table of Cases

Note   The following abbreviations are used:

AC   Law Reports, Appeal Cases
ALJR   Australian Law Journal Reports
All ER   All England Law Reports
BMJ   British Medical Journal
BMLR   Butterworths Medico-Legal Reports
Ch   Law Reports, Chancery Division
Crim LR   Criminal Law Review
CL   Current Law
CMLR   Common Market Law Reports
DLR   Dominion Law Reports
ECR   European Court Reports
Fam   Family Division Law Reports
FLR   Family Law Reports
KB   Law Reports, King's Bench Division
Med LR   Medical Law Reports
Med L Rev.   Medical Law Review
QB   Law Reports, Queen's Bench Division
SC   Session Cases
SJ   Solicitors' Journal
WLR   Weekly Law Reports

Table of Statutes

Statutory instruments

Health circulars

Index

abortion 126, 173
ABPI (Association of the British
Pharmaceutical Industry) 245
accepted practice 10, 15, 83
accident and emergency units 141–3
accountability 12, 17–18, 60–61,
97–8, 114, 234, 239, 240
UKCC Code of Professional
Conduct 41, 43, 44–5
ACHCEW (Association of
Community Health Councils
for England and Wales) 70–71,
72
Action for Victims of Medical
Accidents (AVMA) 59, 63,
71–2, 245
Acts of Parliament see legislation
admission of fault 59
advocacy 15, 70, 100, 101, 107,
114
aggressive patients 178–80
AIDS patients 143
alleged misconduct 49–54, 67
amputation 222
anorexia nervosa 165–6
appeals 54
Association of Community Health
Councils for England and
Wales (ACHCEW) 70–71, 72
Association of the British
Pharmaceutical Industry
(ABPI) 245
assault 235
autonomy 26, 27, 32–3
compulsory care in the community
196–7

constraints on 120
critically ill patients 220
exceptions to the requirement for
informed consent 127–8
informed decisions 122–4
nurses 18
personal flourishing 121, 125–6
social conditioning 124–5, 126
Western society 121–2
AVMA (Action for Victims of Medical
Accidents) 59, 63, 71–2, 245

back injuries 10
battery
blood products 140–41
blood tests 101–2
blood transfusions 106, 109, 120,
121, 208, 209, 212, 222,
223
BMA (British Medical Association) 72
Burns, Dr Tom 181

caesarean section 107–8, 168, 208,
210–11, 223–4
cancer 210, 213, 218, 223, 228
case law 5–6
expert witnesses 10
case studies
critically ill patients
Dr Nigel Cox 203, 204, 216,
226, 227
Tony Bland 199, 202, 203, 211,
212, 215, 225, 227
inadequate resources 141–3, 145–
6, 151–4